DASH DIET

Learn How to Naturally Lower Your Blood Pressure and Lose Weight with an Easy-To-Follow Guide (21-Day Meal Plan Included) + Dash Diet Cookbook with Healthy Low Sodium Recipes

Sheila J. Baker

Table of Contents

DASH DIET FOR BLOOD PRESSURE

*The Complete Guide to Lower Blood Pressure
in Just 14 Days. Change Your Lifestyle by
Following an Effective and Healthy Meal Plan*

Sheila J. Baker

Introduction of Dash Diet for Blood Pressure

In 1996, the Dash diet was discussed in the American Heart Association's annual meeting. A year later, this led to the diet being published in the New England Journal of Medicine for its amazing benefits. After that, further studies were conducted on the Dash diet, resulting in the conclusion that the diet can significantly lower high blood pressure. These are only a handful of the early studies, as time has gone on, more studies have been completed showing the amazing benefits the Dash diet offers. Not only have these studies found the diet to lower blood pressure, but also to reduce cellular DNA damage caused by oxidative stress, lower the risk of cardiovascular diseases, improve bone health, reduce the risk of heart failure, reduce insulin resistance and type II diabetes, and more. A study of the diet completed in 2017 found that if individuals with high blood pressure faithfully follow the Dash diet plan, it could potentially prevent 400,000 deaths caused by cardiovascular disease over ten years.

In short, the Dash diet has been proven to offer powerful, long-lasting, and full-body effects against many of today's most troubling ailments. Whether you have high blood pressure or not, you can likely benefit by implementing this diet in your daily life. You can choose to use this diet to treat high blood pressure, improve overall health and potential life expectancy, or just to lose weight. That is what is great about this plan—it is easy to maintain, full of delicious and balanced meals, can be practiced by a large portion of the population, and it has many benefits.

You may be reading this book because your doctor has told you that you have high blood pressure and need to lower it. However, some people suspect they may have high blood pressure but have not talked about it with their doctor yet. For others, it may simply be a confusing subject, as many people don't explain it in simple everyday terms for the layperson. Let me first say that you should always discuss this with your doctor. If you haven't yet, make an appointment to do so.

When your doctor discusses blood pressure, they may not go into specific or use overly complicated terms. Don't worry, I am here to help! Blood pressure doesn't have to be a confusing subject, you can understand it to come to understand your own health and well-being better. After all, while we must listen to and consult our doctors, we are also our own best advocate, so listen to your body and its needs while also heeding your physician's wise counsel. If you don't trust your doctor, that is okay, you can always try getting a second opinion from another doctor. Thankfully, the subject of blood pressure is pretty straightforward in medical terms, so your doctor will likely have a good handle on the situation. But, if you are uncomfortable seeing a general practitioner regarding your blood pressure and heart health, you may try seeing a cardiologist instead, as they specialize in treating the heart.

Now, one of the most common confusions regarding blood pressure is what the numbers mean. There are two sets of numbers, a top and a bottom one. But, you may be wondering what the difference is and how they impact your health. The top or first number is known as systolic blood pressure. With this number, doctors can determine how much pressure is being pushed against your blood's arteries every time your heartbeats.

The bottom or second number is diastolic blood pressure. While the systolic number measures how much pressure is on your arteries every time the heartbeats, the diagnostic measures how much pressure there is when the heart is at rest between beats.

Because the systolic number measures how much pressure is against your arteries when your heart is at work, this number will be higher and more indicative of risk and disease. While your doctor will keep an eye on both your systolic and diastolic blood pressure, it will be the systolic blood pressure that they are most concerned about, especially in middle age and older adults. As a person ages, their arteries build up plaque and become stiff, which increases the blood flow pressure, thereby increasing the risk of heart attack and disease.

However, while a doctor may focus on the systolic pressure in general, there are exceptions. A high systolic or diastolic number can indicate high blood pressure. Studies have shown that with every 20mm increase in systolic pressure or 10mm in diastolic blood pressure, people experience an increased risk of disease. In fact, for every 20mm or 10mm rise in pressure, a person's risk of death from a heart-related event or stroke doubles for people over the age of forty.

The American Heart Association recognizes five blood pressure ranges, each with their level of risk about heart health. Let's take a look at each, in turn, as if you want to lower your blood pressure with the Dash diet, it is imperative to understand how your blood pressure works, where it is at, and your goal blood pressure range.

Normal

While any reduction in blood pressure is good if you have high blood pressure, your end-goal should get into the normal or safe range. In general, anything under 120mm systolic and 80mm diastolic is considered normal. Having your blood pressure in this range is ideal for your heart health. However, you don't want your blood pressure to go under 90mm systolic and 60mm diastolic, as that is classified as low blood pressure, which causes its own set of problems.

Elevated

Blood pressure is considered elevated when the systolic number is within 120-129mm while the diastolic is no higher than 80mm.

While elevated blood pressure is not yet classified as high blood pressure, people with chronically elevated blood pressure are likely to develop high blood pressure. It is recommended to begin lowering it back to normal now to prevent high blood pressure and its associated risks.

Stage 1, High Blood Pressure

Also known as hypertension, this is the first stage of high blood pressure. During this stage, the systolic number will range between 130mm and 139mm, while the diastolic number will range between 80mm and 89mm. During this high blood pressure stage, your doctor is likely to recommend lifestyle changes, such as the Dash diet, exercise, and other healthy habits. They may even consider adding in blood pressure medication now or shortly if your situation doesn't improve to reduce heart attack and stroke risk.

Stage 2, High Blood Pressure

When a person is in the second stage of hypertension, their blood pressure will regularly maintain a 140mm systolic and 90mm diastolic number, or higher. This stage of high blood pressure is dangerous, and the danger increases, the more the number increases.

At this stage, a doctor is more likely to immediately put their patients on medication and recommend more drastic lifestyle changes. High blood pressure should never be taken lightly, but this is especially true of stage two.

Hypertensive Crisis

When blood pressure gets critically high, it is known as a hypertensive crisis. This is an incredibly dangerous state. Sometimes, it can occur due to acute medical trauma or medical treatment. For instance, someone who has gone into an allergic reaction known as anaphylaxis and been injected with epinephrine to stop the reaction will experience acute high blood pressure. Their blood pressure may spike into a hypertensive crisis until the allergic reaction is under control. The effects of the epinephrine have worn off.

However, some people may have chronic high blood pressure that gets so bad that it reaches a hypertensive crisis. If you reach a hypertensive crisis, wait five minutes, and test your blood pressure again. If your blood pressure is still in this range, then call your doctor immediately and seek medical care. This is vital, as a hypertensive crisis can cause organ damage, shortness of breath, back and chest pains, weakness, difficulty speaking or seeing, and more.

What numbers qualify as a hypertensive crisis? That would be when the systolic number reaches 180mm or higher, and the diastolic number is 120mm.

While the Dash diet's main goal may be to reduce blood pressure, that is not the only goal. Remember, this diet plan has many health benefits, which is why doctors regularly recommend it. One of the great health benefits is that it can help people lose weight.

While this diet is not usually used only for weight loss, you can lose weight as it is a balanced and healthy lifestyle plan. But, at the same time, if you are already at a healthy weight or underweight, you can easily maintain weight as well. This is because you will still largely eat the same foods.

CHAPTER 2:

Overview of the Dash Diet

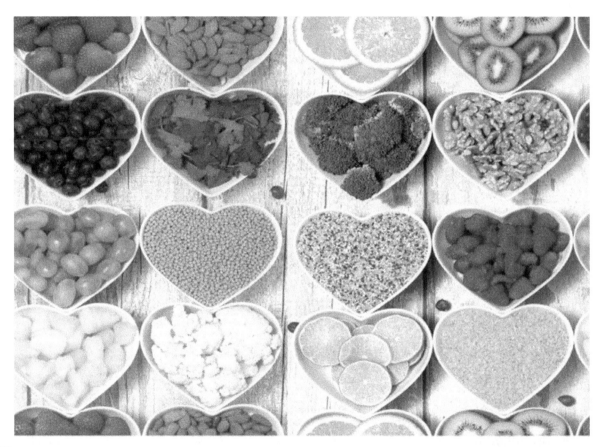

Below you will find a brief overview of the Dash diet to understand this form of nutrition and its principle. Before you jump to the recipes, I strongly recommend that you familiarize yourself with these principles, as it will then be easier for you to put together your recipes and live by them in the future.

What is the Dash Diet?

Dash stands for *Dietary Approaches to Stop Hypertension*. This type of diet is based on research carried out and funded on behalf of the US National Institute of Health (NIH). This research was about determining the role of diet on blood pressure. This diet was created to offer people who suffer from high blood pressure a delicious, tasty, and balanced diet that lowers blood pressure at the same time. This diet is therefore primarily a diet to lower high blood pressure

According to the NIH, the Dash diet promotes healthy eating habits . It shows healthy alternatives to junk food and processed foods. It aims to encourage people to reduce their salt consumption while increasing their calcium, magnesium, and potassium consumption.

Over the years, a number of other studies have proven that the Dash diet is not only effective in lowering blood pressure but that it is also effective in reducing the risk of cardiovascular disease, various cancer diseases, stroke, Diabetes, heart disease, kidney disease, heart failure, and many more diseases.

Although this diet was not developed to reduce body weight, the Dash diet inevitably leads to weight loss solely through the conscious consumption of calories and a diet with healthy foods, which turns out to be another great advantage, especially for overweight hypertensive patients, especially since weight loss is a sensible one Way is to lower blood pressure. With the Dash diet, you can save 2 kilos per week without much effort.

Who is the Dash diet suitable for?

The Dash diet is not a typical diet that briefly changes your diet to achieve a specific goal, such as "losing 10 pounds". The Dash diet is not about restricting yourself for a few days or weeks, but rather a long-term diet change in which a lot of fruit and vegetables, fish and white meat, whole grains and protein-rich foods, high-quality oils, etc., and spices largely replace table salt. Sugar and alcohol are also allowed - but only in very small quantities. So there is no general ban on certain foods; rather, there are more healthy and less unhealthy foods or unhealthy foods are replaced by healthy alternatives.

In this respect, it is suitable for everyone, be it for prevention, to prevent high blood pressure and many diseases such as diabetes, or to naturally regulate blood pressure. Research shows that this type of diet is suitable for adults and children alike.

Concept of the Dash diet

The Dash diet is based on the following principles:

1. Reduction in salt consumption

One of the main goals of the Dash diet is to reduce the consumption of salt drastically.

Of course, man cannot live without salt. The human body contains around 150 to 300 grams of table salt. The amount of salt lost through sweating and other excretions must therefore be replaced. Salt supports bone structure and digestion. It maintains the osmotic pressure in the vessels to maintain the water and nutrient levels. But nowadays our foods are filled with a lot of salt— especially all finished products.

The extent to which increased salt consumption has a negative impact on health is currently the subject of intense discussion among experts, especially since the body excretes excess salt.

But studies from 1970 in Finland already show that too much salt causes blood pressure to skyrocket. It could be shown that the reduced consumption of salt by 30% could even reduce mortality from heart attacks by 80%.

A study on mice published in 2007 at the University Hospital in Heidelberg showed that a lot of salt increases blood pressure: "*Salt promotes the formation of certain messenger substances in the muscles of blood vessels that* cause *the muscle cells to contract. The increased resistance in the blood vessels increases blood pressure.*" Therefore, the Heidelberg scientists,, see considerable advantages in reducing the amount of salt in food compared to conventional drugs.

There is disagreement among scientists about how high the maximum amount of salt can be. While US experts recommend a maximum of 1.5 grams of salt per day, the German Nutrition Society's recommendation is 6 grams per day. The upper limit is 10 grams per day. 6 grams are roughly equivalent to an em teaspoon.

However, this only applies to a healthy person who moves sufficiently and is physically active, and excretes the salt again through sweating. For example, an athlete can tolerate more salt than someone who only moves moderately.

I recommend that you only look at these values as a rough guide and begin to control your salt consumption and gradually reduce it. Also, keep in mind that the maximum amount of salt that you should consume depends on your body constitution and lifestyle.

Recommendation:

- Less is more! Therefore, pay more attention to your salt consumption in the future and reduce it step by step. The keyword is **low-salt, but not salt-free!**

- Avoid finished products (packaged food, pizza, French fries, chips, canned food, various meat and fish products, baked goods, etc.). If necessary, read the list of ingredients.

- If possible, use a **natural salt substitute** (herbs, etc.) in your meals

- Use **low-water cooking methods** such as stewing or steaming. This means that the food remains tastier, and you don't need to salt it as much

2. More vitamin E and minerals

The Dash diet is based on a variety of fruits and vegetables and whole-grain products to provide the body with plenty of vitamins and minerals. Particular attention is paid to minerals such as magnesium and potassium, which help lower or improve blood pressure.

3. More healthy fats and oils

Fats are energy carriers and ensure that fat-soluble vitamins such as vitamins E, D, and K can be absorbed by the body at all. Certain fatty acids, such as omega-3 and omega-6 fatty acids, are also essential, which means that we can only get them from food. Therefore, they should be on a regular meal plan. The **omega-6/3 ratio** plays a vital role in health. Omega-3 fatty acids help to maintain normal blood pressure levels wisely. However, our diet often contains too little omega-3 fatty acids. Good sources of this are **fatty fish** such as herring, mackerel, salmon, and sardines.

This also applies to the use of oils. Z and healthy oils include virgin cold-pressed **olive oil** and **coconut oil** (in organic quality).

Unlike olive oil, coconut oil can also be heated and used for frying and baking. On the other hand, the much-used sunflower oil is less healthy because it only contains omega-6 fatty acids. This creates an imbalance in the omega-3 to omega-6 ratio. A ratio between 1: 2 and 1: 5 should be aimed for.

Ultimately, as with most other diets, the Dash diet should avoid unhealthy fats, especially trans fats, a subgroup of unsaturated fatty acids, and replace them with healthy fats such as those found in nuts, seeds, and fish. Trans fatty acids come from industrial production and are, for example, contained in chips, baked goods, French fries, confectionery, pizza, etc.

4. More fiber

Fiber is an integral part of the Dash diet. A fiber-rich diet, whether through fruits, vegetables, grains, and cereals, positively affects blood pressure and the cardiovascular system.

In contrast to the low carb diet, grain can therefore be consumed. However, it is important to consume only **wholesome grains** (whole grain bread).

5. Egg whites/proteins

Proteins are an important part of the Dash diet and should be consumed in beans, lentils, fish, and soy products.

6. White instead of dark meat

Animal fat should be avoided as far as possible. It is high in cholesterol and saturated fat. Therefore, red meat should be avoided entirely if possible. Instead, white meat (chicken, turkey) can be put on the plate.

7. Avoid butter

Even if opinions differ widely about butter consumption, especially about its effect on the cholesterol level, the Dash diet specifies that butter should be avoided as far as possible. Therefore, butter no longer belongs in the refrigerator. Vegetable oils should serve as a substitute.

Now margarine is anything but healthy and therefore not an alternative in my opinion. Therefore, recommend switching to ghee, the Ayurvedic butter. Ghee is pure butterfat and contains 70% saturated fatty acids. In Ayurveda, Ghee has been used for healing purposes for thousands of years. Studies have shown that **ghee can** even lower cholesterol and prevent diseases such as cardiovascular diseases. The advantage of ghee is that, unlike butter, it can be heated to a high temperature.

8. Low-fat dairy products

The reduced-fat variant should always be preferred for dairy products (max. 1.5% fat content).

9. Less alcohol, caffeine, and nicotine

Alcohol increases blood pressure. The Dash diet recommends avoiding alcohol, beverages containing caffeine, and nicotine as much as possible to reduce blood pressure.

If you don't want to go without your coffee, you should enjoy it with as little or no sugar as possible.

It is also known that smoking increases the risk of heart attacks and strokes. So - if you haven't already done so - put an end to the glowing stick!

10. Reduction of industrial sugar (granulated sugar)

Most people should know by now that too much sugar is not healthy. The Dash diet does not completely exclude sugar. After all, fresh and dried fruits are an important part of this diet, and of course, they also contain sugar (fructose).

What has a negative effect on blood pressure, however, is pure industrial sugar. This can quickly increase blood pressure and should be avoided as far as possible. The best way to regulate daily sugar consumption is to avoid sweets and finished products.

A possible alternative to industrial sugar, which is not exactly cheap, is coconut blossom sugar, which, despite its calories, keeps the blood sugar level more constant.

11. Check daily calorie intake

The Dash diet recommends a calorie intake between 1,500 and 2,300 kcal per day. If you want to lose weight, you should limit the value to 1,500 kcal per day. Of course, this is only a guideline and depends on the basal metabolic rate, age, body weight and size, the muscular mass, gender, and health status. You can find a variety of calculators on the Internet to determine your calorie requirement (e.g., with Fit-for-Fun, Smart Calculator).

CHAPTER 3:

The Health Benefits

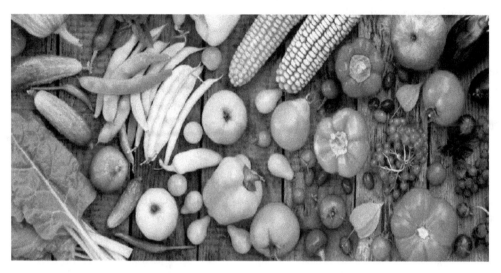

There are many health benefits to this diet, which include the following:

- **Minimizing Hypertension**: It's effective in reducing the sodium content of what you eat, which controls hypertension. Sodium maintains the fluid balance of your body, so high sodium equals hypertension. Less sodium naturally lowers it.

- **Fighting Osteoporosis**: The Dash diet is full of calcium, proteins, and potassium, fighting against the onset of osteoporosis. It helps to prevent the loss of bone strength as well as form.

- **Prevents Cancer:** This diet is rich in antioxidants, which can help to prevent cancer.

- **Reduced Obesity**: If you have a healthy and balanced diet, it activates the metabolism to a sharper ate, which will decompose the stored fat deposits. The dash diet is rich in fibers and low on fat, helping you shed the pounds, especially because exercise is still a must.

- **Improved Heart:** The arteries, valves often cause heart conditions, and veins being clogged with fat, which obstructs the blood flow, and it pressurizes the heart, which can cause a large list of cardiovascular diseases. The Dash diet eradicates the problem by reducing your fat intake, which reduces your risk of heart disease.

- **Preventing Diabetes**: With the Dash diet, you get rid of empty carbs, decreasing the amount of simple sugars found in your blood. This will help you to reduce your risk of diabetes.

- **Helping Kidney Function:** Kidneys are important to maintaining the fluid balance with sodium and potassium. When the balance is disturbed by hypertension, the body holds onto more fluid, causing high blood pressure. The Dash diet can improve the kidney function.

Why It Works

So, you now know the Dash diet's basic benefits, but let's take a deeper look on why the Dash diet truly works.

It's Inclusive

There are few limitations to the diet, and there is every food item available even though some of them do have modifications. There are guides to Dos and Don'ts of this diet and ingredients. Since it's a general diet, it's inclusive to people from most walks of life.

Promotes Exercise

Like most diets that work, this diet does not only focus on food. It promotes physical exercise, as well. With the Dash diet, you get visible results because it stresses daily exercise and routine physical activities. You don't have to overdo the exercise with this diet, but daily exercise is required if you want to trim the fat and help promote heart health.

Proportions

The Dash diet focuses on foods and serving sizes. Balance is key, and it's checked regularly. You must have the correct amount of all ingredients for this diet because nothing is good in excess. Here are the servings that's been determined.

- Grains: 7-8 Daily Servings
- Fruits: 4-5 Daily Servings
- Vegetables: 4-5 Daily Servings
- Low Fat & Fat Free Dairy Products: 2-3 Daily Servings
- Meat, Poultry & Fish: 2 or Less Daily Servings
- Nuts, Seeds & Dry Beans: 4-5 Servings Per Week
- Fats & Oils: 2-3 Daily Servings
- Sweets: Less to 5 Servings per Week

Now you should look at what a serving consists:

- A slice of Bread (Not White Bread)
- 1 Cup of Fruit
- 1 cup of Vegetables
- ½ Cup Cooked Vegetables
- ½ Cup Cooked Fruit
- ½ Cup Cooked Rice
- ½ Cup Cooked Pasta
- 8 Ounces of Milk
- 3 Ounces Cooked Meat
- 3 Ounces Tofu
- 1 Teaspoon Oil

Foods to Have

Here are some foods that you should have, but remember that nothing is good in excess.

- Vegetables
- Fruits
- Poultry
- Seafood
- Seeds
- Pork
- Beef
- No Fat Dairy Products
- Low-Fat Dairy Products
- Nuts
- Grains

Foods to Avoid

You should try to limit these foods as much as possible, and it would be better if you could cut them out of your diet altogether.

- Salt
- High Fat Dairy Products
- Salted Nuts
- Sugary Beverages
- Processed Food
- Animal Based Fats (In Excess)

CHAPTER 4:

Principles of Dash Diet

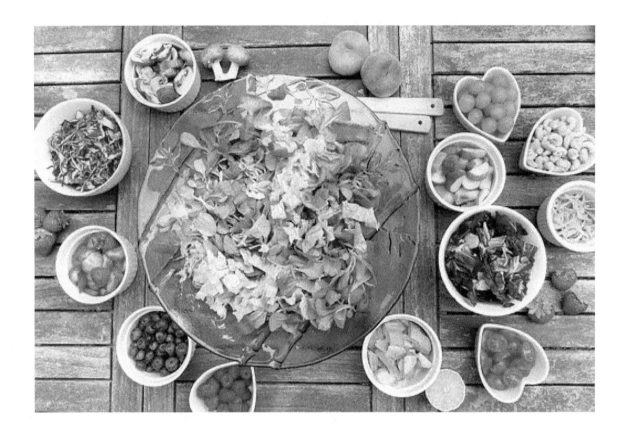

Whole Grains and Starchy Vegetables

Whole grains and starchy vegetables are good sources of fiber, helping to slow glucose absorption in the blood.

Packed with vitamins and minerals, these foods should always be chosen over refined and processed carbohydrates.

Whole grains include brown rice, barley, farro, quinoa, oats, and whole-grain pasta; starchy vegetables include potatoes and sweet potatoes.

Servings: Aim for four to six servings daily. One serving equates to one-half cup of cooked grains, one slice of whole-grain bread, or one medium-sized sweet potato.

Helpful Tips and Tricks: Short on time or don't want to cook? No problem! Instead of making a pot of brown rice, you can look for precooked, frozen whole grains in your grocer's freezer aisle.

Fruits and Vegetables

Fruits and vegetables are a vital part of the Dash diet. Full of vitamins, minerals, and antioxidants, these are nutrient powerhouses in our day-to-day life. These fiber-rich foods help us feel full and satisfied, support lower blood pressure and weight management, and help ward off a variety of diseases. Be sure to eat plenty of alliums, such as garlic, onions, and leeks, as well as a good amount of crucifers, including broccoli, cauliflower, and Brussels sprouts, every week.

Servings: Aim to consume at least four to five servings of vegetables and three fruit servings daily. One serving equates to one-half cup of fruit or cooked vegetables or one cup of raw leafy greens.

Helpful Tips and Tricks: Fresh and frozen will be your go-to foundation, but canned and packed in water, or natural juices are great to keep on hand as a backup option. And don't forget dried fruit, a great addition to your yogurt or oatmeal, or sprinkled on top of a salad!

Building a Plate

Traditional Mediterranean cuisine is enjoyed as part of a balanced lifestyle, including a sustainable approach to eating well. The cornerstone of any healthy diet is a properly proportioned plate. Fruits and vegetables are eaten in plenty, while meats, sweet treats, and wine are enjoyed in moderation. A balanced plate should be one-half non-starchy vegetables, one-quarter whole grains or starchy vegetables, and one-quarter lean protein.

Lean Proteins: Animal and Plant

Lean proteins encompass both animal and plant-based protein sources. In the Dash diet, we place a heavier emphasis on fish and shellfish, with smaller portions of eggs, lean poultry, and meat. When selecting beef, pork, and other animal protein, look for leaner cuts, such as loin and round. These cuts of meat are flavorful and easy to prepare while also being lower in saturated fat. Eggs and poultry are largely excellent choices as well.

Plant-based protein sources are superstars. They are high in fiber and complex carbohydrates while being low in fat. They are also sources of other key minerals and nutrients, such as potassium, magnesium, folate, and iron. Plant-based proteins include beans and legumes, such as lentils, peas, and soy. For our purposes, nuts and seeds will also be part of this category, contributing lean protein and healthy fats.

Servings: Aim to get up to six ounces per day of lean meat, poultry, or seafood. Think of a three-ounce portion as the size of a deck of playing cards. Try to get two to three servings of seafood every week. Aim for four to five servings of nuts, seeds, beans, and legumes per week. One serving is about one-half cup cooked beans or legumes, three ounces of tempeh or tofu, and one-third cup of nuts and seeds.

Helpful Tips and Tricks: Keep low-sodium versions of canned tuna, salmon, and beans on hand to help get meals on the table quickly and easily.

Healthy Fats and Oils

Olives and olive oil are staples in the Dash diet, known for their heart-healthy monounsaturated fat content and anti-inflammatory properties. For more neutral-flavored oil, canola oil is a good choice.

Another great source of healthy fat is avocado. Research has shown that the high levels of oleic acid found in avocados help decrease LDL, the "bad" cholesterol, and boost HDL, the "good" cholesterol.

Servings: Aim for two to three servings of fats and oils daily. One serving equates to one teaspoon of oil or one-quarter of an avocado.

Helpful Tips and Tricks: Making your salad dressing is a great way to incorporate flavorful, low-sodium versions into your daily routine. Use empty jam or nut butter jars to make larger batches, which will keep in the refrigerator for a couple of weeks.

Low-Fat Dairy

Low-fat dairy foods such as cheese and yogurt are foundational foods in the Dash diet. The dairy group contributes important nutrients, including calcium, vitamin D, and potassium. Studies have shown that fermented dairy products, such as yogurt and some cheeses, have an inverse relationship with cardiovascular disease and type 2 diabetes.

There is some evidence that eating fermented dairy foods may help fight inflammation associated with heart disease development.

Servings: Aim to consume two to three servings of low-fat dairy daily. One serving equates to one cup of nonfat or low-fat plain yogurt (includes Greek yogurt) or one-and-a-half ounces of cheese.

Helpful Tips and Tricks: Have a hankering for tuna salad? Use plain yogurt in place of mayonnaise to add protein, flavor, and richness without the added saturated fat and calories. Yogurt can also be added to foods like soup and oatmeal to increase the protein content and add creaminess without using butter or heavy cream.

Limited Added Sugar

The Dash diet naturally decreases sugar intake without making you feel deprived in any way. Dessert and sweet treats can still be part of your weekly routine, but focusing on natural sources of sugar, such as fruit sugars, honey, and maple syrup.

Servings: Aim to limit sugar to five or fewer servings per week. One serving size equals one tablespoon of maple syrup or honey, or one-half cup of ice cream or frozen yogurt.

Helpful Tips and Tricks: Try adding fresh or dried fruit and a teaspoon of jam to a bowl of oatmeal or yogurt in place of sugar.

Limited Sodium

Many foods naturally contain some sodium. However, much of the sodium many of us consume is added to foods, making it too easy for most people to over-consume. You can find it hiding in most processed foods and often added in huge quantities to restaurant meals. Excessive sodium intake is one of the main drivers of high blood pressure.

Using less salt and instead relying on herbs and spices to add bold flavor to foods is a key component of the Dash diet.

Servings: Aim to consume between 1,500 and 2,300 milligrams of sodium per day. For reference, one-quarter teaspoon of kosher salt equals about 500 milligrams of sodium.

Helpful Tips and Tricks: Reach for herbs and spices to create depth of flavor, adding salt in small amounts. You can always add salt, but once it's there you cannot take it away!

The recipes included in the Dash diet follow these guidelines:

Snacks, sides, and desserts: ≤300 milligrams of sodium

Entrées and meals: ≤570 milligrams of sodium

Sneaky Sodium

To keep your sodium intake in check, it is essential to read a food label properly. The first step is to become familiar with portion sizing (i.e., if you eat two servings worth of food, you double your sodium intake). As with sugar, it is important to recognize the difference between naturally occurring sodium in foods and added salt. Some foods, like celery, beets, and milk, organically contain sodium in low levels, which supply our bodies with electrolytes. Added salt is salt added during cooking and processing, and this is what accounts for most of our daily sodium intake. Examples of foods typically loaded with added salt include canned foods, cured and deli-style meats, cheeses, frozen prepared meals, soups, chips, and condiments. To help prevent excessive sodium intake, look for foods labeled "no salt added," "low-sodium," or "sodium-free." When using canned items, such as beans and lentils, rinse well with water before using. And try using garlic, citrus juice, herbs, and spices for flavor before reaching for the saltshaker.

CHAPTER 5:

The Dash Diet and High Blood Pressure

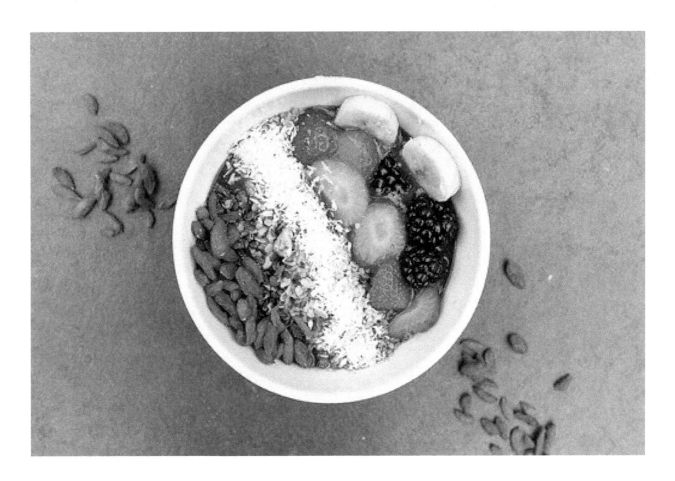

It's estimated that about 50 million people are suffering from high blood pressure in the United States. The actual number is unknown, and it's often called "the silent killer".

The reason is that someone can appear to be completely healthy and yet have high blood pressure.

In many cases, high blood pressure can be due to family history or genetics. However, many environmental causes exist as well, and even if you have a family history, your lifestyle choices may work against you or for you.

Though, the case may be. In other words, you might have a family history but if you don't smoke, maintain your weight, and exercise, you might avoid developing high blood pressure. Conversely, maybe you're relatively healthy even though you have a family history. Adopting an unhealthy lifestyle habit like smoking might tip you over the edge, leading to hypertension.

Some of the most common causes that have been identified include:

- **Smoking:** Cigarette smoking, particularly because people get more nicotine in their system, has been strongly identified as an environmental risk factor for developing high blood pressure.
- **Weight gain/obesity:** Not all overweight people have high blood pressure, but it's clear that being overweight significantly increases your risk of developing it. The heavier you get the higher the risk.
- **Race:** African Americans are more prone to high blood pressure than other groups. However, bear in mind that all racial and ethnic groups have plenty of risk of high blood pressure and its victims include people of all races and from every country across the globe.
- **Kidney disease:** The kidneys are closely tied to the healthy maintenance of blood sugar. They help regulate the amount of fluid and salt in the body. When you are suffering from kidney disease, they may not function as well, and this may lead to fluid and sodium retention, which can cause high blood pressure.
- **Age:** Simply getting older raises risk, although we would never call high blood pressure "normal." However, as you get older, things don't work as well (you knew that, right?). If your joints are stiffening you can bet your arteries are as well. So even though you may be reasonably healthy overall, simply getting older raises your risk of developing some level of high blood pressure. There is some debate about whether older people need to be put under the same standards as to what constitutes a hypertension diagnosis or not, but a general rule applies. You're better off if your blood pressure is below 140/100.
- **Nutritional deficiencies:** By now, you're an expert— nutritional deficiencies of potassium and magnesium can lead to high blood pressure and other health problems like heart palpitations and muscle cramps.
- **Excessive salt in the diet:** We've reviewed this one already – salt causes your body to retain fluid, and it promotes contraction of blood vessels, among other things.

The Dash diet provides an opportunity to address several items on this list. It reduces salt in the diet and addresses the nutritional deficiencies in potassium and magnesium. By consuming large amounts of fruits and vegetables along with a low-fat diet, you'll find that your risk of kidney disease drops as well. Controlling weight can also reduce the risks of developing high blood pressure.

What is Metabolic Syndrome?

We now turn our attention to one of the biggest health problems of the age: *metabolic syndrome*. In many cases, people who have high blood pressure are suffering from metabolic syndrome, and by following the Dash diet, they won't just cure their high blood pressure. They will reset their metabolism and eliminate metabolic syndrome from their lives.

Aside: Your Blood Lipids

Before we formally define metabolic syndrome, we need to review some basics about blood chemistry. The first area we need to review is blood lipids, which are basically the fats flowing around your blood. Kind of gross, huh?

Don't worry, it's all perfectly natural, and you need some level of blood fats. These fats take on a few different forms, some in combination with other molecules. This isn't a chemistry class, so we aren't going to concern ourselves with the gory details, but we need to know what is in your blood and the healthy levels of various components.

Generally, we are concerned with the following:

- Total cholesterol
- LDL cholesterol
- HDL cholesterol
- Triglycerides

No doubt you've heard about total cholesterol already, it's been the medical community's focus for many years. High total cholesterol is associated with an increased risk of developing heart disease and a higher risk of having a heart attack or stroke. In the United States, we measure cholesterol in milligrams of cholesterol per deciliter of blood, or mg/dL. A general rule of thumb is that a total cholesterol of 200 or less is considered low risk, while total cholesterol over 200 is considered an elevated risk, with the risk significantly increasing for each 10 point increase in your total cholesterol. If you consistently show total cholesterol levels of 230 mg/dL or higher, your doctor may want to prescribe statin drugs, which lower cholesterol. Some doctors are more strict than others and will prescribe statins at even lower levels.

Total cholesterol is calculated in the following way:

Total cholesterol = LDL Cholesterol + HDL Cholesterol + 0.20* Triglycerides

You will often see your triglyceride level shown on your blood tests; this means that 20% of your triglyceride level is counted toward your total cholesterol number. Triglycerides are a type of fat that is carried around in your blood.

LDL means Low-Density Lipoprotein. A lipoprotein is a complicated molecule that is made of fat ("lipo") and proteins. Cholesterol is a substance transported through the blood by the LDL or HDL molecule.

LDL is called "bad cholesterol" because it can stick to the walls of your arteries. Over time, they become calcified, and you develop fatty deposits and plaque. The arteries can narrow, eventually causing a heart attack. The LDL cholesterol level in your blood is directly related to the amount of saturated fat you eat per day. An easy way to lower your cholesterol if you're in the borderline range and your doctor isn't putting you on statins yet limits your consumption of saturated fats to 20 grams per day or less. Saturated fat is mostly found in animal products like beef and chicken skin, but it's in all animal products. Dairy and even fish also contain saturated fat. Coconut oil also contains a lot of saturated fat.

HDL is known as "good cholesterol." The reason is that HDL cholesterol is sort of a cleanup crew for the bloodstream. It picks up bad cholesterol, even cleaning it off the artery walls, and it brings it back to the liver. If you have a higher HDL cholesterol (greater than 45 mg/dL, about), you're at lower heart disease risk.

The ratio of total cholesterol to HDL can predict your risk of a heart attack. Generally, you're at lower risk of heart attack if:

Total Cholesterol/HDL < 5

So if someone has total cholesterol of 200 and an HDL cholesterol of 50, their ratio is:

200/50 = 4

This person is considered at low risk of having a heart attack over the next five years. Now suppose someone had total cholesterol of 220 and an HDL cholesterol of 35. Their ratio would be:

220/35 = 6.3

This person is at elevated risk for a heart attack. Their physician may put them on a statin and advise them to take up vigorous aerobic exercise.

While a ratio of less than five is desirable, a ratio of about 3 is considered ideal. While lowering total cholesterol can be achieved with statins, it's not possible to raise HDL with any drugs. A better diet, losing weight, and exercise may raise your HDL.

Although cholesterol is portrayed as a dangerous substance, it's a key component of the body. It's used to build and maintain cell membranes, and it's used to make important hormones in the body. You'd die without any cholesterol. In fact, people with very low cholesterol (below 160) have higher rates of death from all causes.

Triglycerides are also important to measure. High triglycerides indicate a higher risk of heart attack and can cause other problems such as pancreatitis. The ratio of triglycerides to HDL cholesterol is a good indicator of heart attack risk it's better than looking at total cholesterol or even LDL "bad" cholesterol. If the ratio is 1 or less, you're considered to be at low risk of a heart attack. If it's greater than 1, then you're at higher risk.

High LDL cholesterol and a high triglyceride to HDL number not only indicate the risk of heart attack, but they are also a good way to evaluate the risk of stroke. To summarize, it's bad to have:

- High LDL cholesterol
- Low HDL cholesterol
- High triglycerides

Blood Sugar and Insulin

Now we move on from fat to sugar. Like cholesterol, your body needs some sugar in the blood. Without sugar, your brain can't power itself. And just like with cholesterol, when your blood sugar goes too high, serious health problems will result.

The hormone insulin is closely tied to blood sugar. When you eat something, your body begins to digest the carbohydrates in the food you ate. They are broken down into glucose, the simplest form of sugar or starch that there is. The glucose then enters your bloodstream.

The cells of your body need glucose for energy and your brain needs it to survive. However, the cells of the body aren't just going to suck up the glucose. They need a trigger, to be told to take it up. That trigger is provided by insulin. Think of insulin as a key fitting into the cell's door and opening it so that the glucose can go inside and leave the bloodstream.

In a normal, healthy person, this process works fine. A healthy person could eat a plate of spaghetti. About two hours later, their blood sugar would be about 140 mg/dL (we measure blood sugar in the same units used to measure cholesterol).

CHAPTER 6:

Your Dash Diet Primer

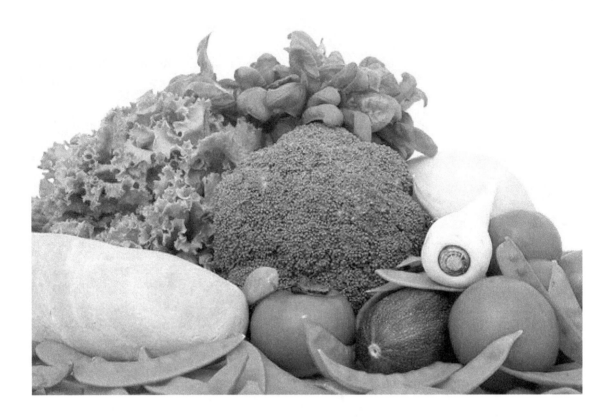

The Dash diet represents a balanced, varied eating style that offers you a practical nutrition solution to help you move toward your goals. Healthy eating is complicated by all of the fad diets and trends in the world. We are going to ignore that and focus on a style of eating that you can feel confident in. Here, we will take a closer look at why the Dash diet is so different and better than what you may be used to.

From the Standard American Diet to the Dash Diet

The average American's diet needs some improvement. Health concerns such as obesity, diabetes, and hypertension have become more of a norm than an exception. According to the 2013–2014 data from the National Health and Nutrition Examination Survey, more than two-thirds of the American population was considered either overweight or obese. This is partially due to a disconnect between the amount of calories we consume from food, the amount our bodies need, and the amount we expend through physical activity. What's much more concerning is the reality that approximately one in three American adults has high blood pressure, also known as hypertension, which is one of the most significant risk factors for cardiovascular disease. This does not even mention that so few of us consume adequate amounts of the most healthful foods like fruits and vegetables.

This is where the Dietary Approaches to Stop Hypertension (Dash) eating style, which was developed and tested specifically to address the pervasive issue of high blood pressure, or hypertension, comes in. First unveiled in an article in *The New England Journal of Medicine* in 1997, the Dash diet has grown in mainstream popularity and was ranked as the number one Best Diet for Healthy Eating by the *U.S. News & World Report* in 2018, which also ranked it number four on the list of easiest diets to follow.

How Dash Diet Aids in Weight Loss and Lowers Blood Pressure

The Dash diet is highlighted by its inclusion of ample fruits, vegetables, and low-fat dairy products while being generally low in saturated fat.

The Dash diet's blood pressure lowering qualities are often attributed to it being naturally high in potassium, calcium, and magnesium, which are found abundantly in the diverse array of foods that the diet incorporates.

In 2001, the Dash group conducted a follow-up study to the one published in 1997. It again published their results in *The New England Journal of Medicine*.

The study found the Dash diet was even more effective at lowering blood pressure when combined with dietary sodium restriction. Excessive sodium, or salt, has since become well known to increase some people's risk of hypertension.

Changes to diet while also restricting sodium have become recognized as effective in lowering blood pressure. These Dash diet trials and many others that followed effectively proved that the Dash diet can significantly reduce your blood pressure.

But how does the Dash dietary pattern stack up for those who may be trying to lose weight? From my perspective as a registered dietitian, the Dash diet offers you the opportunity to shed unwanted pounds in a practical and nonrestrictive way.

For example, the Dash diet contains plenty of fruits and whole grains, which many common diets restrict. It focuses on balanced and moderate inclusion of all different types of foods.

With that in mind, it comes as no surprise that a 2016 review study published in the *Obesity Reviews* journal concluded that the "Dash diet is a good choice for weight management, particularly for weight reduction in overweight and obese participants."

Caloric Intake on the Dash Diet

The Dash diet guidelines center on the inclusion of various food groups in amounts that vary based on individual characteristics.

These food groups and their recommended serving sizes are determined by personal characteristics, including your age, gender, and activity level. Before you can determine your Dash diet guidelines, you need to estimate your calorie needs.

The first two tables below will help you estimate your body's daily caloric needs. To figure out your estimated daily calorie intake, take a look at your physical activity.

Sedentary is defined as little to no physical activity, **moderately active** as walking 1½ to 3 miles a day plus light physical activity, and **active** as exercising at the level suggested by the 28-day plan that follows.

Estimated Daily Calorie Needs for Women

AGE (YEARS)	SEDENTARY	MODERATELY ACTIVE	ACTIVE
19–30	2,000	2,100	2,400
31–50	1,800	2,000	2,200
51+	1,600	1,800	2,100

Estimated Daily Calorie Needs for Men

AGE (YEARS)	SEDENTARY	MODERATELY ACTIVE	ACTIVE
19–30	2,400	2,700	3,000
31–50	2,200	2,500	2,900
51+	2,000	2,300	2,600

Keep in mind that if your goal is to reduce your body weight, a simple first step is to consume approximately 250 to 500 calories fewer than what the above tables estimate.

Please consult the charts below, which you can then use with the Daily Serving Recommendations table to determine your approximate serving recommendations for each food group. With that in mind, I want you to worry less about the actual number of calories you are aiming for and more about what this means in terms of total daily servings in the Dash diet.

Estimated Daily Calorie Needs for Women Who Want to Lose Weight

AGE (YEARS)	SEDENTARY	MODERATELY ACTIVE	ACTIVE

19–30	1,500–1,750	1,600–1,850	1,900–2,150
31–50	1,300–1,550	1,500–1,750	1,700–1,950
51+	1,100–1,350	1,300–1,550	1,600–1,850

Estimated Daily Calorie Needs for Men Who Want to Lose Weight

AGE (YEARS)	SEDENTARY	MODERATELY ACTIVE	ACTIVE
19–30	1,900-2,150	2,200–2,450	2,500–2,750
31–50	1,700-1,950	2,000–2,250	2,400–2,650
51+	1,500-1,750	1,800–2,050	2,100–2,350

The Dash Diet Guidelines

It is important to identify the different kinds of foods that the Dash diet encourages you to consume. There are some general guidelines for eating in a Dash -friendly way. You should limit sodium, sweets, sugary drinks, and red meat that you consume. But how and why? Let's discuss the different kinds of foods you should be consuming and why they help improve your health.

Whole Grains and Starchy Vegetables

Let's face it: Almost all of us love carbohydrate-rich foods, and although very-low-carb diets may help some lose weight in the short term, they aren't particularly sustainable and certainly not very enjoyable. The Dash diet doesn't suggest avoiding carbs; it suggests you enjoy the most fiber- and nutrient-dense versions of them, which is a message I can certainly get behind. Brown rice, quinoa, whole-grain bread, whole-grain pasta, and potatoes (any variety) are Dash-approved.

Serving size: 1 slice whole-grain bread, ½ cup brown rice or quinoa, 1 medium-size potato or sweet potato.

VEGETABLES

Vegetables are, simply put, the most important part of any eating style. The high potassium content of most vegetables—especially leafy greens—plays an important role in blood pressure regulation. Your kidneys play an important role in blood pressure management by controlling the fluid balance in your body. Your sodium and potassium intake further modify this balance. Most people consume much more sodium than potassium, which affects your kidneys' ability to control your blood pressure properly. This balance can be restored in most people by increasing potassium intake and decreasing sodium intake. Vegetables contain a vast amount of other healthful nutrients and antioxidant compounds. From a weight-management perspective, the high fiber content of vegetables promotes satiety and may prevent weight gain. A 2009 study in *The Journal of Nutrition* found that women who increased their fiber intake tended to gain less weight and body fat over time. Most Americans simply do not eat enough fiber, with only about half the population consuming the American Heart Association's recommended daily target goal of 30 grams per day.

Serving size: ½ cup cooked veggies like broccoli or Brussels sprouts, 1 cup raw vegetables like spinach.

Fruit

Sometimes popular "diets" suggest eliminating fruit because it contains moderate amounts of natural sugars. If this is something you've heard, I want you to ignore that sentiment and embrace fruit as a very healthy component of the Dash diet and a critical part of longevity and good health.

Besides being absolutely delicious, fruit is rich in potassium, fiber, and other important nutrients that help support both blood pressure and weight management.

Serving size: 1 medium-size piece of fruit like an apple or banana, ½ cup fruit like blueberries or strawberries.

Low-Fat Dairy and Alternatives

Dairy products and alternatives are an important part of the Dash eating plan for a few reasons. The high calcium content of these foods is thought to play an important role in blood-pressure regulation because it modifies the hormones responsible for the tension in your blood vessels. The high protein content also supports weight management and weight loss because protein not only makes us feel full but requires extra energy for our bodies to break down. This largely explains why studies, including a 2015 review published in *The American Journal of Clinical Nutrition*, tend to find that adequate protein intake is usually associated with better outcomes in managing both our weight and our appetite.

Serving size: 1 cup skim milk, 1 cup 0% yogurt (including Greek), 1 cup soy milk, 1½ ounces skim cheese.

Lean Meat, Poultry, Fish, and Alternatives

These are dietary staples for many and important contributors of protein and magnesium in the Dash diet. Anyone who happens to be vegan or vegetarian knows that you can confidently replace animal-protein sources listed here with legume-based protein such as tofu, lentils, chickpeas, and others. When selecting meat, leaner cuts like tenderloin, sirloin, or eye of round for beef are optimal as they contain less fat than other commonly available varieties. Avoiding purchasing cuts with visible fat or trimming fat before cooking also helps. We suggest consuming multiple servings of fish per week.

Serving size: 1 ounce of cooked meat, poultry, or fish, 1 egg, 3 ounces of tofu

Nuts, Seeds, and Legumes

This group of foods is unique for the simple fact they are among the relatively small group of plant-based foods that contain both iron and protein, which are two of the important nutrients animal proteins offer us. Unlike most meat types, though, these choices are high in fiber and heart-healthy monounsaturated fat while also being much lower in saturated fat.

Serving size: ⅓ cup raw or unsalted nuts or seeds, 2 tablespoons nut butter, ½ cup cooked legumes (preferably cooked from raw, not canned, which are higher in sodium).

CHAPTER 7:

Hypertension

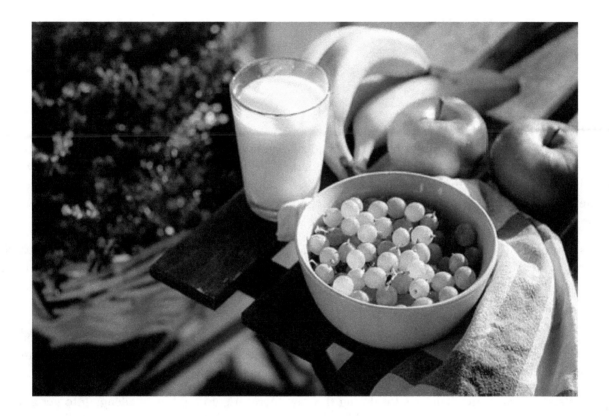

Hypertension is high blood pressure. Blood pressure measures blood pressure, contrary to the arterial walls as the heart pumps blood through your body. Blood pressure is read with two numbers. For instance, a reading of 120/80 or below is known as normal blood pressure. The first number or numerator is the systolic blood pressure. The next number or denominator is the diastolic blood pressure.

When the blood pressure is above 140/90, it is considered high blood pressure. When the blood pressure reads above 120/80 but significantly less than 140/90, it is considered pre-hypertension. Pre-hypertension will likely result in hypertension.

Causes of Hypertension

There are multiple reasons why a person might develop high blood pressure. Some reasons are:

- An excessive amount of sodium in the torso because of a sodium-rich diet
- The underlying condition of the nervous system, kidneys, or arteries
- Hormonal imbalance

- Age
- Obesity
- Overconsumption of alcohol
- Genealogy of hypertension
- Diabetes
- Smoking
- Adrenal gland disorders
- Preeclampsia in pregnancy
- Some medications
- Renal artery stenosis
- Hyperparathyroidism

Symptoms of Hypertension

Most hypertension cases go unnoticed by the individual experiencing high blood pressure because there are rarely outward symptoms. People only normally understand they have high blood pressure whenever they go to the doctor and have their blood pressure checked. Devoid of your blood pressure checked regularly is quite dangerous. This is also true as a person ages because hypertension can result in cardiovascular disease or kidney issues while being unacquainted with the high blood pressure issue.

Many symptoms of a hazardous disease referred to as malignant hypertension include severe headaches, vomiting, nausea, convulsion, vision changes, and nosebleeds. When you have these symptoms, go right to an ER.

Testing for Hypertension

Your doctor will need your blood pressure reading many times before diagnosing you with hypertension. Multiple readings taken at differing times of day are then averaged to diagnose high blood pressure.

A person's blood pressure changes a lot during the day; therefore, it could be challenging to get a precise reading of actual high blood pressure. Your blood pressure is usually lowest when you initially get up each day and may increase as much as 30% during the day because of fluctuations in hormones, activity, stress levels, and eating. You can even purchase a blood pressure monitor to consider your blood pressure reading at home. Your medical provider can help you with what monitors are best and how exactly to utilize them properly. In the home, you may take your blood pressure at precisely the same time every day to discover if you will find fluctuations within the readings. This will supply the most accurate estimate of if your blood pressure is decreasing or increasing because of lifestyle changes.

Let's face it; hypertension is no joke. You will find serious risks connected with uncontrolled high blood pressure that may lead to disability and death. The glad tidings are that hypertension is preventable and treatable with lifestyle changes.

How Many People in the USA Have problems with Hypertension?

The current statistics show that roughly one in three American adults have problems with high blood pressure. That is approximately 65 million people. Half of most Americans older than 60 now have hypertension. The chance of the American having high blood pressure sometime in his/her life is approximately 90%.

Those statistics are not very good odds. However, the good news is the fact that prevention and delay of high blood pressure are possible.

Complications of Hypertension

Danger to the heart

- The heart is in charge of blood flow through the entire body, but high blood pressure can create serious problems because of this vital organ.
- Coronary artery disease limits the blood circulation towards the heart. This may lead to a heart attack.
- An enlarged left heart may result from high blood pressure forcing the heart to work too much. At these times, the left side of the heart thickens and stiffens. This may lead to a heart attack, heart failure, or sudden death.
- Heart failure could be caused by any risk of strain of elevated blood pressure around the heart muscle. This may cause the heart to be overwhelmed and fail.

Danger to the brain

The brain needs a healthy way to obtain nourishing blood to be able to work correctly.

- The transient ischemic attack can be called a mini-stroke. It is a short disruption within the blood circulation to the mind, often the effect of a blood clot because of high blood pressure. A TIA often warns of the impending full stroke.
- Heatstroke occurs when the brain does not obtain the oxygen and nutrients it needs to operate properly. This causes the mind cells to die. High blood pressure damages and weakens the brain's arteries, which could result in a stroke.
- Dementia is an illness of the mind that may cause issues with speaking, thinking, memory, movement, and vision. Although there are many factors behind dementia, one primary cause may be narrowing the arteries resulting in the brain due to high blood pressure. Even high blood pressure that begins at age can lead to later dementia.
- Mild cognitive impairment may be the stage between regular brain function changes that occurs because of aging and much more severe problems like Alzheimer's. That is due to blocked blood circulation with the arteries because of high blood pressure damage.

Danger to the arteries

Arteries are elastic, flexible, and strong.

They provide your body with nutrients and oxygen. Increased pressure because of high blood pressure can cause various issues for the arteries.

- Arteriosclerosis may be the thickening and narrowing of arteries that may occur due to high blood pressure. This may reduce blood circulation to vital organs, like the heart, brain, kidneys, lungs, and arms. Arteriosclerosis could cause an array of problems, including chest pain, heart attack, heart stroke, kidney and heart failure, and eye damage.
- An Aneurysm is a bulge inside the artery due to high blood pressure. The aneurysm can rupture, causing internal bleeding that may result in death.

Danger to the eyes

The eyes are given blood by tiny arteries that are often damaged by high blood pressure.

- Eye blood vessel damage could be due to high blood pressure. This can result in retina damage and bleeding in the eyes, blurry vision, and total lack of vision.
- Fluid buildup beneath the retina is undoubtedly due to leaking arteries beneath the retina. This may result in impaired vision.
- Harm to the optic nerve is normally due to blocked blood circulation for the optic nerve, killing nerve cells in the attention, resulting in bleeding in the focus and vision loss.

Danger to the kidneys

The kidneys will be the body's filtering. The filtration process depends on healthy arteries. High blood pressure can hinder the filtration procedure and can result in many kinds of kidney disease.

- Kidney failure can occur when high blood pressure causes harm to the arteries that result in the kidneys and the tiny blood vessels in the kidneys. This damage could make kidneys work less effectively, filtering waste and will bring about waste accumulation.
- Kidney scarring or due to scaring for the glomeruli, which are clusters of arteries in the kidneys. These scars make it impossible for the kidneys to filter waste, which may result in kidney failure.
- Aneurysm towards the kidney arteries can be caused by harm to the arteries resulting in the kidneys. High blood pressure causes this damage.

Sexual dysfunction

Sexuality is usually crucial in maintaining lasting relationships. Sexual dysfunction can result in anxiety and troubles in personal relationships.

- Male sexual dysfunction could be due to high blood pressure since it damages the arteries and arteries that limit the blood circulation towards the penis. This helps it be increasingly difficult to accomplish or maintain an erection.
- Female sexual dysfunction because of high blood pressure is due to limited blood circulation for the sexual organs, resulting in decreased libido, dryness, and difficulties reaching orgasm.

Other issues linked to high blood pressure are;

- Bone loss could be due to increased calcium levels being excreted in the urine due to high blood pressure.
- Sleep problems, for example, sleep apnea, are typical in about 50% of most people with high blood pressure issues.

The potential risks of hypertension far outweigh the momentary pleasure in continuing to consume a "typical American diet." Unfortunately, most Americans lack proper nutritional education to improve their lifestyle. By reading this book, you are making the first positive step toward a wholesome life.

CHAPTER 8:

Phase One- Reset Your Metabolism in Two Weeks

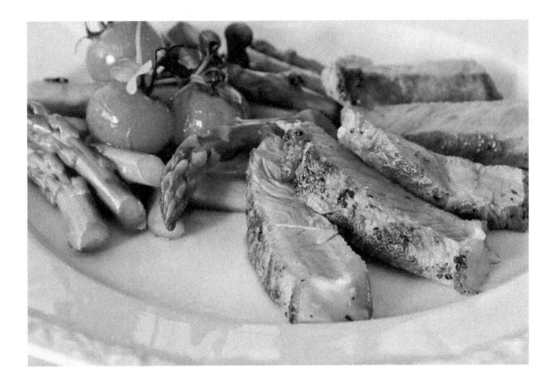

Now, it's time to get into the nitty-gritty of actually implementing the diet. For the first week, we'll keep things fairly simple and restrict portions. The purpose of this is two-fold. First off, we don't want to be overwhelmed with details when starting the new diet, so we'll offer very simple meal suggestions for the first seven days to help you get started.

Second, we'll limit portions a little bit for the second 7 days, so that you can get going with weight loss. However, the meals we suggest should be pretty satisfying for most people, so they won't leave you feeling hungry.

Meat shopping list

- Salmon
- Trout
- Canned sardines
- Skinless + Boneless chicken breasts
- Skinless + Boneless chicken thighs
- 85% lean ground beef or ground turkey
- Pork loin
- Eggs

- Smoked salmon

Beans and Legumes

- 3 cans of garbanzo beans
- 1 can kidney beans
- Lentils
- Peanuts

Nuts and seeds

- Pre-packed Planters heart-healthy nut mix, eat one bag per day.
- Unsalted walnuts
- Unsalted pumpkin seeds
- Unsalted almond or walnut butter

Dairy

- Grass-Fed Whole milk
- Swiss cheese
- Parmesan cheese
- Unsweetened yogurt

Fruits and vegetables

- Spinach (no limits to greens)
- Arugula
- Tomatoes
- Onions
- Garlic
- Strawberries
- Blackberries
- Blueberries
- Raspberries
- Bananas (great source of potassium)
- Avocados
- Spring mix
- Apples
- Cucumbers
- Bell peppers
- Asparagus
- Celery
- Kale

Whole-grains

- Whole wheat pasta
- Whole grain bread
- Wild rice
- Brown rice
- Steel-cut oats
- Quinoa

Oils and dressings

- Extra-Virgin Olive oil
- Avocado oil
- Olive or Avocado based mayo
- Low sodium mustard
- Vinegar
- Olive oil and vinegar salad dressing
- Balsamic vinegar salad dressing
- Any low or no-sodium spices (cumin, basil, cayenne pepper, lemon pepper, garlic powder, thyme, etc.)

A 14 Day Reset

Exercise suggestions:

- 30-minute walk, five days per week
- Swimming
- Cycling
- Jogging
- Mountain biking
- Walk the dog daily
- Hiking on mountain or nature trails
- Elliptical
- Rowing machine
- Pilates
- Yoga

Getting enough sleep is another thing that people don't get enough of, like drinking water. To maintain good health, it's a good idea to keep your sleep rhythms relatively constant and to get a good 6-8 hours of sleep per night. Everyone is different, so for some folks getting only 6 hours of sleep can be more than sufficient, while others will be dragging. Make sure that you get the amount of sleep that works best for you.

Stress reduction is important as well. When you're under chronic stress, whether it's worrying about work problems, being unable to pay bills or marital problems, your health suffers. It turns out that being constantly stressed can increase levels of inflammation throughout the body. If you're looking into adopting the Dash diet, then you're looking to improve your health. While what you put in your mouth is certainly very important, don't neglect what's going on in your mental life either. The body works in a feedback loop with the brain, and when you're feeling a lot of stress, the body reacts.

Sometimes stress is over events or situations we don't have immediate control over if we can control it. Maybe you have a large credit card debt that is hard to pay off right now. Rather than sitting around stressed out about it constantly – which accomplishes nothing – you should focus on your health instead. One good suggestion is to take up yoga twice a week. Although we listed yoga as an exercise activity —and it is— yoga is also great for promoting relaxation and reducing stress. You can also add a daily meditation or prayer session to your day. If possible, do that first thing in the morning. People with young children at home or who face a long commute may find that difficult, but you can find some small time frame of 5-10 minutes a day where you can meditate and relax to help relieve stress. Deep breathing exercises throughout the day can help as well.

With many diets, starting a new diet can create stress with friends and family, particularly if you are living with one or more people in your home who don't share your desire to embark on a new diet. The good thing about the Dash diet is that it isn't all that radical, so it shouldn't be too hard to get family members to go along. Eating out isn't too problematic either since many of the top options listed in this diet are available in most restaurants. One thing you can do is request no salt versions of a dish, and certainly avoid using the salt shaker.

You can also request that the cook not use MSG on your meal, and substitute vegetables for unacceptable side items. Salmon is a popular item in just about any restaurant these days – but beware of high salt sauces, particularly teriyaki sauce.

The only restaurants that might cause you trouble are Chinese and Japanese. If possible, ask for low-sodium soy sauce.

It's also essential to keep a good attitude and forgive yourself when you make transgressions on a diet – which are inevitable on occasion. Using the example we just talked about, you might get a craving for Chinese food, or coworkers might drag you along for sushi. It's not going to be the end of the world if you eat one meal with high salt content.

Rather than beating yourself up over it, go along and enjoy it and make up for it later. That is the beauty of this diet it's very adaptable.

Let's just say that, for example, you end up eating sushi, which will mean eating a lot of salt. Obviously, you can be very strict on the following day to make up for it, but you can also make up for it at your next meal.

- At your next meal, eat very low salt, as low as possible.

- Include items that will help keep everything in balance. Add a full avocado, for example.

- Eat some fruit which has zero or low sodium but lots of potassium, like an apple or an orange.

- Drink some extra water to help flush your system.

There is no need to be neurotic about it. As you can see from these suggestions moving on from mistakes is relatively easy. Another transgression people often face having to eat sweets. Maybe you're at a birthday party. Do you want to be the annoying curmudgeon who is always talking about their special diet? Probably not –so you'll probably just take the piece of cake they offer you. Again, don't sweat it. If you get into a situation where you consume a lot of sweets:

- Count the cake as your five servings of sweets for the week, and don't eat anymore.

- At your next meal, reduce your carbs a bit and up your fat and protein intake instead. Substitute avocado or extra fish for some whole grains to temporarily reduce your carbs.

- Go fruitless for a day, and just get by eating seven or eight servings of vegetables. Opt for low carb vegetables like stir-fried spinach.

- Plan ahead. You'll digest sweets like cake and ice cream better by getting a good dose of fat beforehand. So if you have the choice, eat higher fat and low carb dish for your main meal before eating something like cake.

Finally, don't skip meals. The premise behind the Dash diet is to be satisfied. That is one reason why fat is so important on the diet. Fat helps you feel satiated.

When you're satiated, you eat less overall. That's why calorie counting isn't used on a Dash diet. While the Dash diet is more portion based, it also avoids counting calories.

Suggested 14-Day Meal Plan for Phase One

Our suggestion for the first seven days is to keep it simple. Getting bogged down in complicated recipes may make it hard to adjust to your new diet while you're busy with all the other activities of life.

Day One

Breakfast: Hard-boiled egg, 1-2 slices Canadian bacon, 6 oz. Tomato juice.

Lunch: Crazy Japanese Potato and Beef Croquettes

Mid-afternoon snack: 4 oz. light yogurt, 10 cashews

Dinner: Healthy Avocado Beef Patties

Snack: pepper strips, 1/4 cup guacamole

Day Two

Breakfast: Open-Faced Breakfast Sandwich

Lunch: Lovely Faux Mac and Cheese

Mid-afternoon snack: 1 stick light cheese, cherry tomatoes

Dinner: Bulgur Appetizer Salad

Snack: Coconut-mint bars

Day Three

Breakfast: Mini Egg Beaters omelet, 4-6 oz. tomato juice

Lunch: 2-3 Turkey Swiss roll-ups, 1/2 to 1 cup coleslaw, raw snow peas or sugar snap peas

Mid-afternoon snack: 1 stick light cheese, baby carrots

Dinner: Roasted sliced turkey, sautéed carrots and onions

Snack: 10 peanuts

Day Four

Breakfast: Cinnamon Oatmeal

Lunch: Epic Mango Chicken

Mid-afternoon snack: The Delish Turkey Wrap

Dinner: Green Egg Scramble

Snack: Cocoa Bars

Day Five

Breakfast: Scrambled eggs, 1-2 slices Canadian bacon, 4-6 oz. diet cranberry juice

Lunch: Cold fried chicken breast, coleslaw, baby carrots

Mid-afternoon snack: 4 oz. light yogurt, 1 oz. almonds

Dinner: Super savory sliders, 1 cup broccoli, side salad with balsamic dressing

Snack: vanilla biscuits

Day Six

Breakfast: Egg White and Vegetable Omelet

Lunch: Chicken and Cabbage Platter

Mid-afternoon snack: Strawberry Buckwheat Pancakes

Dinner: Spiced Scramble

Snack: Cinnamon Apple Chips

Day Seven

Breakfast: Turkey Swiss roll-up, 4-6 oz. tomato juice

Lunch: Salad with grilled chicken

Mid-afternoon snack: 1 light cheese stick, celery sticks

Dinner: 1/4 rotisserie chicken, 1 cup frozen peas

Snack: 6 baby carrots

Day Eight

Breakfast: Fruity Green Smoothie

Lunch: Hearty Chicken Liver Stew

Mid-afternoon snack: Chilled Strawberry & Walnut Porridge

Dinner: Chicken rolls with pesto

Snack: 10 peanuts

Day Nine

Breakfast: Lemon Zucchini Muffins

Lunch: Stir Fried Green Beans

Mid-afternoon snack: Cocoa Bars

Dinner: Almond Butternut Chicken

Snack: Cinnamon Apple Chips

Day Ten

Breakfast: Blueberry Breakfast Quinoa

Lunch: Chicken Quesadilla

Mid-afternoon snack: 4 oz. light yogurt, 1 oz. almonds

Dinner: Spicy Pumpkin Seeds Bowls

Snack: 4 oz light yogurt, 18 cashews

Day Eleven

Breakfast: Fruity Green Smoothie

Lunch: Juicy and Peppery Tenderloin

Mid-afternoon snack: Pepper strips, 1/4 cup guacamole

Dinner: Ravaging Beef Pot Roast

Snack: Strawberry and Nut Granola

Day Twelve

Breakfast: Blueberry-Maple Oatmeal

Lunch: Mustard Chicken

Mid-afternoon snack: Fruit & Nut Granola

Dinner: Coconut Curry Cauliflower Soup

Snack: Apple and Pecans Bowls

Day Thirteen

Breakfast: Greek-Style Breakfast Scramble

Lunch: Duck with Cucumber and Carrots

Mid-afternoon snack: Cinnamon Apple Chips

Dinner: Hearty Chicken Liver Stew

Snack: 1 light cheese stick, celery sticks

Day Fourteen

Breakfast: Lemon Zucchini Muffins

Lunch: Chicken and Carrot Stew

Mid-afternoon snack: Fruit & Nut Yogurt Crunch

Dinner: Shrimp Muffins

Snack: 4 oz. Light yogurt, 1 oz. almonds

CHAPTER 9:

Phase Two

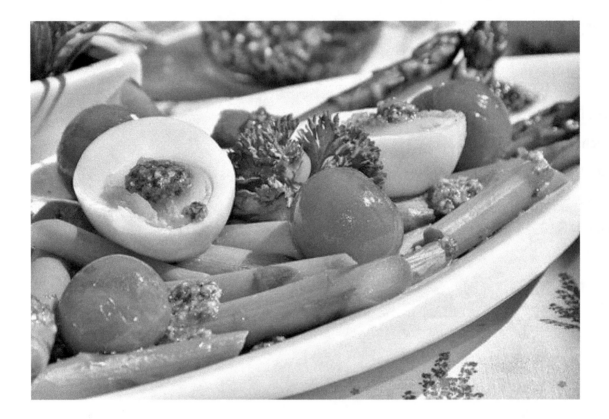

In phase two of the diet, which can begin after the first two weeks, we want to ramp up our servings. In phase 2, we will add all the healthy food options you want to include in the diet and form the foundation for a long-term future of health.

Transitioning to Phase Two

For phase two, we'll use the following recommendations.

Dairy

- Begin making sure that you include 2-3 moderate servings per day of dairy. This can include more than one serving of milk (1/2 cup per serving), a ½ cup of cottage cheese, a ½ cup of unsweetened yogurt, and cheese in 1.5-ounce portions eaten as a snack or used for your recipes.

- If you're lactose intolerant try lactose-free milk or substitute almond or hemp milk.

- Whole milk from grass-fed cows is generally recommended.

- If you drink coffee, you can add a bit of half-and-half if you prefer cream in your coffee.

Nuts and Seeds

- In phase two, you should eat at least one serving of nuts per day, and you can eat more if your appetite demands it. The key is to avoid overeating. So if you're satisfied, don't eat more. If you eat lunch and are still hungry, then eat ¼ cup of nuts.

Starchy vegetables

- Limit starchy vegetables like sweet potatoes, potatoes, turnips, and yams to at most one serving per day.

Fruits

- Our suggestion is to consume adequate fruits, but don't overdo it. While the standard Dash diet allows up to five servings per day, we recommend that you limit your consumption to three servings per day on this diet. It's important to recognize that on the Dash Mediterranean solution diet, since you're consuming a lot more fat than you would on the Dash diet alone, you should cut back somewhere else. Cutting back on fruit is a good place to cut because while the fruit is generally healthy, it does contain a lot of sugar, which will be problematic for some people. You can get all the nutrients you get out of fruits like apples, kiwis, and oranges elsewhere. One possible substitute is a quarter or a half-cup of berries, which have a lower glycemic index and lower carb content than large fruits like apples and bananas. You can also get many vitamins, minerals, antioxidants, and phytonutrients that you get from fruits by consuming large amounts of leafy green vegetables.

- Eat your avocados. The potassium and magnesium in avocados help regulate blood pressure. Monounsaturated fats help make you feel satisfied while promoting heart health. In addition, remember that avocados contain large amounts of fiber that can help with digestive issues.

Proportions and Foods for Phase Two

- 7 servings per day of vegetables, only one of which is a starchy vegetable.

- 3 servings per day of fruit, one of which is an avocado. Also, substitute berries for large sugary fruits.

- 6 servings per day of whole grains. We're cutting back to make room for fat consumption.

- 2-3 moderately sized servings of dairy.

- 2-3 servings of meat (count eggs as meat).

- Olive oil is unlimited. Consume as much as you want to feel satisfied.

- You can introduce some sweets in phase two if desired. Do you need sweets? You might find that if you abandon sweets after some time passes, you rarely crave them.

Sample 7-Day Meal Plan for Phase Two

Day One
Breakfast: Greek-Style Breakfast Scramble

Lunch: The Delish Turkey Wrap

Mid-afternoon snack: Fruit & Nut Crunch

Dinner: Zucchini Bowls

Snack: Spicy Pumpkin Seeds Bowls

Day Two
Breakfast: Blueberry Green Smoothie

Lunch: Almond butternut Chicken

Mid-afternoon snack: Cocoa Bars

Dinner: Juicy and Peppery Tenderloin

Snack: Apple and Pecan Bowls

Day Three
Breakfast: Green Smoothie

Lunch: Zucchini Zoodles with Chicken and Basil

Mid-afternoon snack: Strawberry & Nut Granola

Dinner: Fascinating Spinach and Beef Meatballs

Snack: Fruit & Nut Yogurt Crunch

Day Four
Breakfast: Fruit and Yogurt Breakfast Salad

Lunch: Duck with Cucumber and Carrots

Mid-afternoon snack: Cinnamon Apple Chips

Dinner: Hearty Chicken Liver Stew

Snack: 1 light cheese stick, celery sticks

Day Five

Breakfast: Spiced Scramble

Lunch: Parmesan Baked Chicken

Mid-afternoon snack: Strawberry Buckwheat Pancake

Dinner: Lovely Faux Mac and Cheese

Snack: Vanilla Biscuits

Day Six

Breakfast: Cheesy Baked Eggs

Lunch: Healthy Avocado Beef Patties

Mid-afternoon snack: Strawberry Buckwheat Pancakes

Dinner: Mustard Chicken

Snack: 6 baby carrots

Day Seven

Breakfast: Green Egg Scramble

Lunch: Crazy Japanese Potato and Beef Croquettes

Mid-afternoon snack: Strawberry & Nut Granola

Dinner: Ravaging Beef Pot Roast

Snack: 10 peanuts

CHAPTER 10:

Breakfast

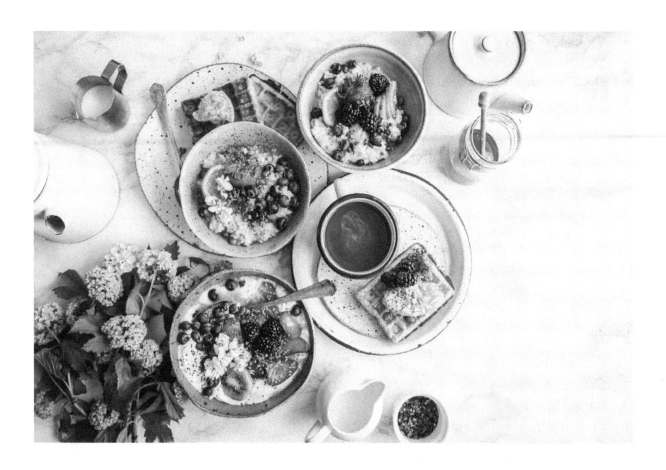

Open-Faced Breakfast Sandwich

- **Preparation time: 10 minutes**
- **Cooking time: 7 minutes**
- **Servings: 1**

Ingredients:

- ½ Whole-wheat English muffin
- 1 slice Reduced-fat (2%) Swiss cheese
- Olive oil cooking spray
- ½ cup unseasoned egg whites
- 1 ½ tsp. green part only finely chopped scallion

Directions:

1. Toast the English muffin in the broiler.
2. Turn off the broiler, top the muffin with cheese pieces and let stand until cheese melted, about 30 seconds. Transfer to a plate.
3. Meanwhile, spray a skillet with oil and heat over medium-high heat.
4. Add the egg whites and cook. Tilt the pan so the mixture spreads on the pan.
5. Use a spatula to lift the edges to cook well.
6. Fold the edges of the egg mixture to make a patty.
7. Transfer the egg patty to the muffin and sprinkle with scallion.
8. Serve.

Nutrition:

- Calories: 166
- Fat: 2g
- Carb: 17g
- Protein: 21g
- Sodium 350mg

Cinnamon Oatmeal

- **Preparation time: 10 minutes**
- **Cooking time: 4 minutes**
- **Servings: 1**

Ingredients:

- 2 cups Low-fat milk
- 1 ½ tsp. Vanilla extract
- 1 1/3 cups quick oats
- ¼ cup Light brown sugar
- ½ tsp. Ground cinnamon

Directions:

1. Add milk and vanilla to a saucepan and bring to a boil.
2. Then reduce heat, stir in oats, brown sugar, and cinnamon, and cook and stir for 3 minutes.
3. Serve.

Nutrition

- Calories: 208
- Fat: 3g
- Carb: 59g
- Protein: 8g
- Sodium: 58mg

Egg White and Vegetable Omelet

- **Preparation time: 10 minutes**
- **Cooking time: 20 minutes**
- **Servings: 1**

Ingredients:

- 6 Egg whites
- 1 Tbsp. Water
- 2 tsp. Olive oil
- ½, Yellow onion chopped
- 1, Tomato diced
- 2 asparagus stalks cut into small pieces
- 3 to 4 Mushrooms sliced

Directions

1. Whisk egg whites in a bowl. Add 1 tbsp. water, and whisk until well blended.
2. Heat 1 tsp. oil in a skillet. Add tomato, onion, asparagus, mushrooms, and sauté until vegetables are tender for about 3 to 4 minutes. Remove from pan and set aside.
3. Add another tsp. of oil and heat for 2 minutes.
4. Add beaten eggs to the pan, tilting the pan to cover the entire pan.
5. Cook until eggs are almost finished but still soft in the middle.
6. Add vegetable mixture to the middle of the omelet. Fold and serve.

Nutrition

- Calories: 145
- Fat: 4.5g
- Carb: 19g
- Protein: 8.5g
- Sodium: 77mg

Fruity Green Smoothie

- **Preparation time: 5 minutes**
- **Cooking time: 0 minutes**
- **Servings: 1**

Ingredients:

- 2 cups Fresh spinach leaves –
- 1 peeled Medium banana –,
- Strawberries – 8, trimmed
- Orange juice - ½ cup
- Crushed ice – 1 cup

Directions:

1. Blend everything in a blender.
2. Serve.

Nutrition:

- Calories: 235
- Fat: 1.5g
- Carb: 56g
- Protein: 5g
- Sodium: 64mg

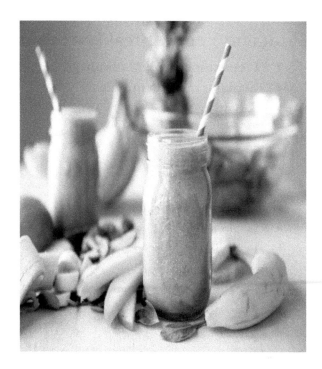

Fruit and Yogurt Breakfast Salad

- **Preparation time: 10 minutes**
- **Cooking time: 15 minutes**
- **Servings: 6**

Ingredients:

- 2 cups Water
- ¼ tsp Salt
- ¾ cup Quick-cooking brown rice
- ¾ cup Bulgur
- 1 cored and chopped large apple
- 1 cored and chopped large pear
- 1 peeled and cut Orange
- 1 cup dried cranberries
- 8 ounces low-fat or nonfat Greek-style yogurt, plain

Directions:

1. Heat water in a large pot.
2. Add salt, rice, and bulgur to boiling water. Lower heat to low.
3. Cover, and simmer for 10 minutes. Remove from heat.
4. Transfer grains to a large bowl and keep in the refrigerator until chilled.
5. Remove chilled grains from the refrigerator.
6. Add apple, pear, oranges, and dried cranberries.
7. Fold in the yogurt and mix gently until grains and fruit are mixed well.
8. Serve.

Nutrition:

- Calories: 190
- Fat: 1g
- Carb: 40g
- Protein: 4g
- Sodium: 118mg

Blueberry Breakfast Quinoa

- **Preparation time: 10 minutes**
- **Cooking time: 15 minutes**
- **Servings: 4**

Ingredients:

- 2 cups Low-fat nonfat milk
- 1 cup Quinoa
- ¼ cup Honey
- ½ tsp. Cinnamon
- ¼ cup Chopped almonds, pecans, or walnuts
- ½ cup Fresh blueberries

Directions:

1. Add milk in a saucepan, and bring to a low boil. Add quinoa and return to boil. Cover.
2. Simmer (on low heat) until most of the liquid is absorbed, about 12 to 15 minutes. Remove from heat.
3. Stir remaining ingredients into quinoa, cover, and allow to stand for 10 minutes more.
4. Serve.

Nutrition:

- Calories: 320
- Fat: 5g
- Carb: 59g
- Protein: 12g
- Sodium: 70mg

Blueberry-Maple Oatmeal

- **Preparation time: 10 minutes**
- **Cooking time: 7 minutes**
- **Servings: 1**

Ingredients:

- ½ cup (old-fashioned style) rolled oats
- ½ cup Nonfat milk
- Pinch of sea salt
- 1 Tbsp. Chia seeds
- 2 tsp. Maple syrup
- 2 cups Fresh blueberries

Directions:

1. In a bowl, combine oats, milk, and salt. Cover and place in the refrigerator overnight.
2. Before serving, top with chia seeds, maple syrup, and blueberries.

Nutrition:

- Calories: 260
- Fat: 4g
- Carb: 49g
- Protein: 9g
- Sodium: 160mg

Lemon Zucchini Muffins

- **Preparation time: 10 minutes**
- **Cooking time: 7 minutes**
- **Servings: 1**

Ingredients:

- 2 cups all-purpose flour
- ½ cup Sugar
- 1 Tbsp. Baking powder
- ¼ tsp. Salt
- ¼ tsp. Cinnamon
- ¼ tsp. Nutmeg
- 1 cup shredded zucchini
- ¾ cup Nonfat milk
- 2 Tbsp. Olive oil
- 2 Tbsp. Lemon juice
- 1 Egg
- Nonstick cooking spray

Directions:

1. Preheat the oven to 400F. Grease the muffin tins.
2. Combine sugar, flour, baking powder, salt, cinnamon, and nutmeg in a bowl.
3. In another bowl, combine zucchini, milk, oil, lemon juice, and egg. Stir well.
4. Add zucchini mixture to flour mixture. Stir until just combined.
5. Pour batter into prepared muffin cups.
6. Bake for 20 minutes and serve.

Nutrition:

- Calories: 145
- Fat: 4g
- Carb: 25g
- Protein: 3g
- Sodium: 62mg

Greek-Style Breakfast Scramble

- **Preparation time: 10 minutes**
- **Cooking time: 8 minutes**
- **Servings: 1**

Ingredients:

- Nonstick cooking spray
- 1 cup fresh spinach
- ½ cup Mushrooms
- ¼ Onion
- 1 Whole egg
- 2 Tbsp. Feta cheese
- Freshly ground black pepper to taste

Directions:

1. Heat a skillet over medium heat.
2. Spray with cooking spray and add spinach, mushrooms, and onion.
3. Sauté for 2 to 3 minutes or until onions turn translucent and spinach has wilted
4. Meanwhile, whisk egg and egg whites together in a bowl. Add feta cheese and pepper.
5. Pour egg mixture over vegetables.
6. Cook eggs, stirring with a spatula, for 3 to 4 minutes, or until eggs are cooked.
7. Serve.

Nutrition:

- Calories: 150
- Fat: 7g
- Carb: 6g
- Protein: 17g
- Sodium: 440mg

Blueberry Green Smoothie

- **Preparation time: 10 minutes**
- **Cooking time: 0 minutes**
- **Servings: 2**

Ingredients:

- 2 cups Chopped mixed greens
- ¼ cup Water–
- 1/3 cup Chopped carrot
- ½ cup Frozen blueberries
- ½ cup Chopped unpeeled cucumber
- ¼ cup Unsweetened almond milk
- 4 Ice cubes

Directions

1. Place the greens and water in a blender. Blend until smooth.
2. Add the remaining ingredients and blend until desired consistency is achieved.
3. Serve.

Nutrition:

- Calories: 82
- Fat: 1g
- Carb: 17g
- Protein: 4g
- Sodium: 66mg

Green Smoothie

- **Preparation time: 5 minutes**
- **Cooking time: 0 minutes**
- **Servings: 2**

Ingredients:

- 2 cups Spinach
- 2 chopped Large kale leaves
- ¾ cup Water
- 1 large, chopped Frozen banana
- ½ cup Frozen mango
- ½ cup Frozen peach
- 1 Tbsp. Ground flaxseeds
- 1 Tbsp. Almond butter

Directions:

1. Place the spinach, kale, and water in the blender.
2. Blend until smooth.
3. Then add fruit, flaxseeds, and nut butter and blend until smooth.
4. Serve.

Nutrition:

- Calories: 157
- Fat: 2g
- Carb: 35g
- Protein: 5g
- Sodium: 48mg

Ravaging Beef Pot Roast

- **Preparation time: 10 minutes**
- **Cooking time: 75 minutes**
- **Servings: 4**

Ingredients:

- 3 ½ pounds beef roast
- 4 ounces mushrooms, sliced
- 12 ounces beef stock
- 1 onion soup mix
- ½ cup Italian dressing, low sodium, and low fat

Directions:

1. Take a bowl and add the stock, onion soup mix, and Italian dressing.
2. Stir.
3. Put beef roast in a pan.
4. Add mushrooms, stock mix to the pan, and cover with foil.
5. Preheat your oven to 300 degrees F.
6. Bake for 1 hour and 15 minutes.
7. Let the roast cool.
8. Slice and serve.
9. Enjoy with the gravy on top!

Nutrition:

- Calories: 700
- Fat: 56g
- Carbohydrates: 10g
- Protein: 70g
- Sodium: 350mg

Cheesy Baked Eggs

- **Preparation Time: 5 minutes**
- **Cooking time: 15 minutes**
- **Servings: 4**

Ingredients:

- 4 large eggs
- 75g (3oz) cheese, grated
- 25g (1oz) fresh rocket (arugula) leaves, finely chopped
- 1 tablespoon parsley
- ½ teaspoon ground turmeric
- 1 tablespoon olive oil

Directions:

1. Grease each ramekin dish with a little olive oil.
2. Divide the rocket (arugula) between the ramekin dishes, then break an egg into each one.
3. Sprinkle a little parsley and turmeric on top, then sprinkle on the cheese.
4. Place the ramekins in a preheated oven at 220C/425F for 15 minutes, until the eggs are set, and the cheese is bubbling.

Nutrition:

- Calories: 198
- Fat: 9g
- Fiber: 3g
- Carbs: 2g
- Protein: 13g
- Sodium: 45mg

Green Egg Scramble

- **Preparation Time: 10 minutes**
- **Cooking time: 5 minutes**
- **Servings: 1**

Ingredients:

- 2 eggs, whisked
- 25g (1oz) rocket (arugula) leaves
- 1 teaspoon chives, chopped
- 1 teaspoon fresh basil, chopped
- 1 teaspoon fresh parsley, chopped
- 1 tablespoon olive oil

Directions:

1. Mix the eggs with the rocket (arugula) and herbs.
2. Heat the oil in a frying pan and pour it into the egg mixture.
3. Gently stir until it's lightly scrambled. Season and serve.

Nutrition:

- Calories 250
- Fat: 5g
- Fiber: 7g
- Carbs: 8g
- Protein: 11g
- Sodium: 70mg

Spiced Scramble

- **Preparation Time: 10 minutes**
- **Cooking time: 5 minutes**
- **Servings: 1**

Ingredients:

- 25g (1oz) kale, finely chopped
- 2 eggs
- 1 spring onion (scallion) finely chopped
- 1 teaspoon turmeric
- 1 tablespoon olive oil
- Sea salt
- Freshly ground black pepper

Directions:

1. Crack the eggs into a bowl.
2. Add the turmeric and whisk them. Season with salt and pepper.
3. Heat the oil in a frying pan, add the kale and spring onions (scallions) and cook until it has wilted.
4. Pour in the beaten eggs and stir until eggs have scrambled together with the kale.

Nutrition:

- Calories: 259
- Fat: 3g
- Fiber: 4g
- Carbs: 3g
- Sodium: 30mg
- Protein: 9g

Strawberry Buckwheat Pancakes

- **Preparation Time: 20 minutes**
- **Cooking time: 5 minutes**
- Servings: 4

Ingredients:

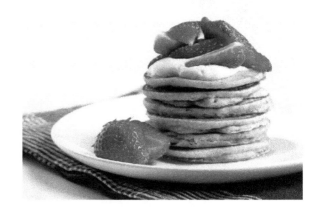

- 100g strawberries, chopped
- 100g buckwheat flour
- 1 egg
- 250mls milk
- 1 teaspoon olive oil
- 1 teaspoon olive oil for frying
- Freshly squeezed juice of 1 orange
- 175 calories per serving

Directions:

1. Pour the milk into a bowl and mix in the egg and a teaspoon of olive oil.
2. Sift in the flour to the liquid mixture until smooth and creamy.
3. Allow it to rest for 15 minutes. Heat a little oil in a pan and pour in a quarter of the mixture (or the size you prefer.)
4. Sprinkle in a quarter of the strawberries into the batter.
5. Cook for around 2 minutes on each side.
6. Serve hot with a drizzle of orange juice.
7. You could try experimenting with other berries such as blueberries and blackberries

Nutrition:

- Calories: 106
- Fat: 2g
- Sodium: 79mg
- Fiber: 10g
- Carbs: 7g
- Protein: 8g

CHAPTER 11:

Lunch

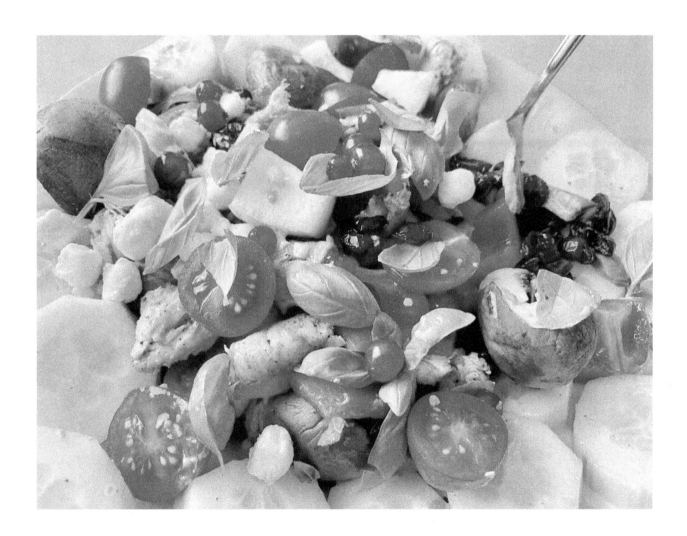

Fascinating Spinach and Beef Meatballs

- **Preparation time: 10 minutes**
- **Cooking time: 20 minutes**
- **Servings: 2**

Ingredients:

- ½ cup onion
- 4 garlic cloves
- 1 whole egg
- ¼ teaspoon oregano
- Pepper as needed
- 1 pound lean ground beef
- 10 ounces spinach

Directions:

1. Preheat your oven to 375 degrees F.
2. Take a bowl and mix in the rest of the ingredients, and using your hands, roll into meatballs.
3. Transfer to a sheet tray and bake for 20 minutes.
4. Enjoy!

Nutrition:

- Calorie: 200
- Fat: 8g
- Carbohydrates: 5g
- Protein: 29g
- Sodium: 350mg

Juicy and Peppery Tenderloin

- **Preparation time: 10 minutes**
- **Cooking time: 20 minutes**
- **Servings: 2**

Ingredients:

- 2 teaspoons sage, chopped
- Sunflower seeds and pepper
- 2 1/2 pounds beef tenderloin
- 2 teaspoons thyme, chopped
- 2 garlic cloves, sliced
- 2 teaspoons rosemary, chopped
- 4 teaspoons olive oil

Directions:

1. Preheat your oven to 425 ° F.
2. Take a small knife and cut incisions in the tenderloin; insert one slice of garlic into the incision.
3. Rub meat with oil.
4. Take a bowl and add sunflower seeds, sage, thyme, rosemary, pepper and mix well.
5. Rub the spice mix over tenderloin.
6. Put rubbed tenderloin into the roasting pan and bake for 10 minutes.
7. Lower temperature to 350 degrees F and cook for 20 minutes more until an internal thermometer reads 145 degrees F.
8. Transfer tenderloin to a cutting board and let sit for 15 minutes; slice into 20 pieces and enjoy!

Nutrition:

- Calorie: 183
- Fat: 9g
- Carbohydrates: 1g
- Protein: 24g
- Sodium: 30mg

Healthy Avocado Beef Patties

- **Preparation time: 15 minutes**
- **Cooking time: 10 minutes**
- **Servings: 2**

Ingredients:

1. 1 pound 85% lean ground beef
2. 1 small avocado, pitted and peeled
3. Fresh ground black pepper as needed

Directions:

1. Pre-heat and prepare your broiler to high.
2. Divide beef into two equal-sized patties.
3. Season the patties with pepper accordingly.
4. Broil the patties for 5 minutes per side.
5. Transfer the patties to a platter.
6. Slice avocado into strips and place them on top of the patties.
7. Serve and enjoy!

Nutrition:

- Calories: 568
- Fat: 43g
- Net Carbohydrates: 9g
- Protein: 38g
- Sodium: 33mg

Lovely Faux Mac and Cheese

- **Preparation time: 15 minutes**
- **Cooking time: 45 minutes**
- **Servings: 2**

Ingredients:

- 5 cups cauliflower florets
- Sunflower seeds and pepper to taste
- 1 cup coconut almond milk
- ½ cup vegetable broth
- 2 tablespoons coconut flour, sifted
- 1 organic egg, beaten
- 1 cup cashew cheese

Directions:

1. Preheat your oven to 350 ° F.
2. Season florets with sunflower seeds and steam until firm.
3. Place florets in a greased ovenproof dish.
4. Heat coconut almond milk over medium heat in a skillet; make sure to season the oil with sunflower seeds and pepper.
5. Stir in broth and add coconut flour to the mix, stir.
6. Cook until the sauce begins to bubble.
7. Remove heat and add beaten egg.
8. Pour the thick sauce over the cauliflower and mix in cheese.
9. Bake for 30-45 minutes.
10. Serve and enjoy!

Nutrition:

- Calories: 229
- Fat: 14g
- Carbohydrates: 9g
- Protein: 15g
- Sodium: 150mg

Epic Mango Chicken

- **Preparation time: 25 minutes**
- **Cooking time: 10 minutes**
- **Servings: 2**

Ingredients:

- 2 medium mangoes, peeled and sliced
- 10-ounce coconut almond milk
- 4 teaspoons vegetable oil
- 4 teaspoons spicy curry paste
- 14-ounce chicken breast halves, skinless and boneless, cut into cubes
- 4 medium shallots
- 1 large English cucumber, sliced and seeded

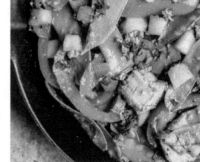

Directions:

1. Slice half of the mangoes and add the halves to a bowl.
2. Add mangoes and coconut almond milk to a blender and blend until you have a smooth puree.
3. Keep the mixture on the side.
4. Take a large-sized pot and place it over medium heat, add oil, and allow the oil to heat up.
5. Add curry paste and cook for 1 minute until you have a nice fragrance.
6. Add shallots and chicken to the pot and cook for 5 minutes.
7. Pour mango puree into the mix and allow it to heat up.
8. Serve the cooked chicken with mango puree and cucumbers.
9. Enjoy!

Nutrition:

- Calories: 398
- Fat: 20g
- Carbs: 32g
- Protein: 26g
- Sodium: 320mg

Chicken and Cabbage Platter

- **Preparation time: 9 minutes**
- **Cooking time: 14 minutes**
- **Servings: 2**

Ingredients:

- ½ cup sliced onion
- 1 tablespoon sesame garlic-flavored oil
- 2 cups shredded Bok-Choy
- 1/2 cups fresh bean sprouts
- 1 1/2 stalks celery, chopped
- 1 ½ teaspoons minced garlic
- 1/2 teaspoon stevia
- 1/2 cup chicken broth
- 1 tablespoon coconut aminos
- 1/2 tablespoon freshly minced ginger
- 1/2 teaspoon arrowroot
- 2 boneless chicken breasts, cooked and sliced thinly

Directions:

1. Shred the cabbage with a knife.
2. Slice onion and add to your platter alongside the rotisserie chicken.
3. Add a dollop of mayonnaise on top and drizzle olive oil over the cabbage.
4. Season with sunflower seeds and pepper according to your taste.
5. Enjoy!

Nutrition:

- Calories: 368
- Fat: 18g
- Protein: 42g
- Fiber: 3g
- Carbs: 11g
- Sodium: 150mg

Mustard Chicken

- **Preparation time: 10 minutes**
- **Cooking time: 40 minutes**
- **Servings: 2**

Ingredients:

- 2 chicken breasts
- 1/4 cup chicken broth
- 2 tablespoons mustard
- 1 1/2 tablespoons olive oil
- 1/2 teaspoon paprika
- 1/2 teaspoon chili powder
- 1/2 teaspoon garlic powder

Directions:

1. Take a small bowl and mix mustard, olive oil, paprika, chicken broth, garlic powder, chicken broth, and chili.
2. Add chicken breast and marinate for 30 minutes.
3. Take a lined baking sheet and arrange the chicken.
4. Bake for 35 minutes at 375 degrees F.
5. Serve and enjoy!

Nutrition:

- Calories: 531
- Fat: 23g
- Carbs: 10g
- Protein: 64g
- Sodium: 250mg

Chicken and Carrot Stew

- **Preparation time: 15 minutes**
- **Cooking time: 6 minutes**
- **Servings: 2**

Ingredients:

- 4 boneless chicken breast, cubed
- 3 cups of carrots, peeled and cubed
- 1 cup onion, chopped
- 1 cup tomatoes, chopped
- 1 teaspoon of dried thyme
- 2 cups of chicken broth
- 2 garlic cloves, minced
- Sunflower seeds and pepper as needed

Directions:

1. Add all of the listed ingredients to a Slow Cooker.
2. Stir and close the lid.
3. Cook for 6 hours.
4. Serve hot and enjoy!

Nutrition:

- Calories: 182
- Fat: 3g
- Carbs: 10g
- Protein: 39g
- Sodium: 120mg

Almond Butternut Chicken

- **Preparation time: 15 minutes**
- **Cooking time: 30 minutes**
- **Servings: 2**

Ingredients:

- ½ pound Nitrate free bacon
- 6 chicken thighs, boneless and skinless
- 2-3 cups almond butternut squash, cubed
- Extra virgin olive oil
- Fresh chopped sage
- Sunflower seeds and pepper as needed

Directions:

1. Prepare your oven by preheating it to 425 degrees F.
2. Take a large skillet and place it over medium-high heat, add bacon and fry until crispy.
3. Take a slice of bacon and place it on the side, crumble the bacon.
4. Add cubed almond butternut squash in the bacon grease and sauté, season with sunflower seeds and pepper.
5. Once the squash is tender, remove skillet and transfer to a plate.
6. Add coconut oil to the skillet and add chicken thighs, cook for 10 minutes.
7. Season with sunflower seeds and pepper.
8. Remove skillet from stove and transfer to oven.
9. Bake for 12-15 minutes, top with the crumbled bacon and sage.
10. Enjoy!

Nutrition:

- Calories: 323
- Fat: 19g
- Carbs: 8g
- Protein: 12g
- Sodium: 130mg

Zucchini Zoodles with Chicken and Basil

- **Preparation time: 10 minutes**
- **Cooking time: 10 minutes**
- **Servings: 2**

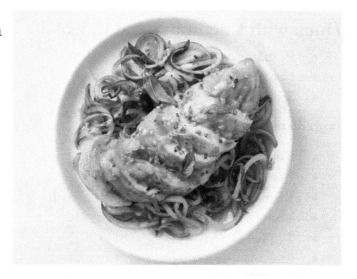

Ingredients:

- 2 chicken fillets, cubed
- 2 tablespoons ghee
- 1 pound tomatoes, diced
- ½ cup basil, chopped
- ¼ cup almond milk
- 1 garlic clove, peeled, minced
- 1 zucchini, shredded

Directions:

1. Sauté cubed chicken in ghee until no longer pink.
2. Add tomatoes and season with sunflower seeds.
3. Simmer and reduce liquid.
4. Prepare your zucchini Zoodles by shredding zucchini in a food processor.
5. Add basil, garlic, coconut almond milk to the chicken and cook for a few minutes.
6. Add half of the zucchini Zoodles to a bowl and top with creamy tomato basil chicken.
7. Enjoy!

Nutrition:

- Calories: 540
- Fat: 27g
- Carbs: 13g
- Protein: 59g
- Sodium: 180mg

Duck with Cucumber and Carrots

- **Preparation time: 9 minutes**
- **Cooking time: 14 minutes**
- **Servings: 2**

Ingredients:

- 1 duck, cut up into medium pieces
- 1 chopped cucumber, chopped
- 1 tablespoon low sodium vegetable stock
- 2 carrots, chopped
- 2 cups of water
- Black pepper as needed
- 1 inch ginger piece, grated

Directions:

1. Add duck pieces to your Instant Pot.
2. Add cucumber, stock, carrots, water, ginger, pepper, and stir.
3. Lock up the lid and cook on LOW pressure for 40 minutes.
4. Release the pressure naturally.
5. Serve and enjoy!

Nutrition:

- Calories: 206
- Fats: 7g
- Carbs: 28g
- Protein: 16g
- Sodium: 20mg

Parmesan Baked Chicken

- **Preparation time: 5 minutes**
- **Cooking time: 20 minutes**
- **Servings: 2**

Ingredients:

- 2 tablespoons ghee
- 2 boneless chicken breasts, skinless
- Pink sunflower seeds
- Freshly ground black pepper
- ½ cup mayonnaise, low fat
- ¼ cup parmesan cheese, grated
- 1 tablespoon dried Italian seasoning, low fat, low sodium
- ¼ cup crushed pork rinds

Directions:

1. Preheat your oven to 425 ° F.
2. Take a large baking dish and coat it with ghee.
3. Pat chicken breasts dry and wrap with a towel.
4. Season with sunflower seeds and pepper.
5. Place in baking dish.
6. Take a small bowl and add mayonnaise, parmesan cheese, Italian seasoning.
7. Slather mayo mix evenly over chicken breast.
8. Sprinkle crushed pork rinds on top.
9. Bake for 20 minutes until topping is browned.
10. Serve and enjoy!

Nutrition:

- Calories: 850
- Fat: 67g
- Carbs: 2g
- Protein: 60g
- Sodium: 120mg

Crazy Japanese Potato and Beef Croquettes

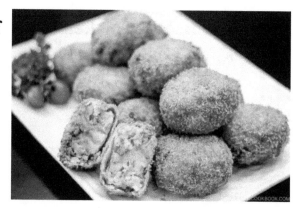

- **Preparation time: 10 minutes**
- **Cooking time: 20 minutes**
- **Servings: 2**

Ingredients:

- 3 medium russet potatoes, peeled and chopped
- 1 tablespoon almond butter
- 1 tablespoon vegetable oil
- 3 onions, diced
- ¾ pound ground beef
- 4 teaspoons light coconut aminos
- All-purpose flour for coating
- 2 eggs, beaten
- Panko bread crumbs for coating
- ½ cup oil, frying

Directions:

1. Take a saucepan and place it over medium-high heat; add potatoes and sunflower seeds water, boil for 16 minutes.
2. Remove water and put potatoes in another bowl, add almond butter and mash the potatoes.
3. Take a frying pan and place it over medium heat, add 1 tablespoon oil and let it heat up.
4. Add onions and stir fry until tender.
5. Add coconut aminos to beef to onions.
6. Keep frying until beef is browned.
7. Mix the beef with the potatoes evenly.
8. Take another frying pan and place it over medium heat; add half a cup of oil.
9. Form croquettes using the mashed potato mixture and coat them with flour, then eggs and finally breadcrumbs.
10. Fry patties until golden on all sides.
11. Enjoy!

Nutrition:

- Calories: 239
- Fat: 4g
- Carbs: 20g
- Protein: 10g
- Sodium: 70mg

Spicy Chili Crackers

- **Preparation time: 15 minutes**
- **Cooking time: 60 minutes**
- **Servings: 20**

Ingredients:

- ¾ cup almond flour
- ¼ cup coconut four
- ¼ cup coconut flour
- ½ teaspoon paprika
- ½ teaspoon cumin
- 1 ½ teaspoons chili pepper spice
- 1 teaspoon onion powder
- ½ teaspoon sunflower seeds
- 1 whole egg
- ¼ cup unsalted almond butter

Directions:

1. Preheat your oven to 350 degrees F.
2. Line a baking sheet with parchment paper and keep it on the side.
3. Add ingredients to your food processor and pulse until you have a nice dough.
4. Divide dough into two equal parts.
5. Place one ball on a sheet of parchment paper and cover with another sheet; roll it out.
6. Cut into crackers and repeat with the other ball.
7. Transfer the prepped dough to a baking tray and bake for 8-10 minutes.
8. Remove from oven and serve.
9. Enjoy!

Nutrition:

- Carbs: 2.8g
- Fiber: 1g
- Protein: 1.6g
- Fat: 4.1g
- Sodium: 70mg

Golden Eggplant Fries

- **Preparation time: 10 minutes**
- **Cooking time: 15 minutes**
- **Servings: 2**

Ingredients:

- 2 eggs
- 2 cups almond flour
- 2 tablespoons coconut oil, spray
- 2 eggplant, peeled and cut thinly
- Sunflower seeds and pepper

Directions:

1. Preheat your oven to 400 ° F.
2. Take a bowl and mix with sunflower seeds and black pepper.
3. Take another bowl and beat eggs until frothy.
4. Dip the eggplant pieces into the eggs.
5. Then coat them with the flour mixture.
6. Add another layer of flour and egg.
7. Then, take a baking sheet and grease with coconut oil on top.
8. Bake for about 15 minutes.
9. Serve and enjoy!

Nutrition:

- Calories: 212
- Fat: 15.8g
- Carbs: 12.1g
- Protein: 8.6g
- Sodium: 120mg

Traditional Black Bean Chili

- **Preparation time: 10 minutes**
- **Cooking time: 4 hours**
- **Servings: 2**

Ingredients:

- 1 ½ cups red bell pepper, chopped
- 1 cup yellow onion, chopped
- 1 ½ cups mushrooms, sliced
- 1 tablespoon olive oil
- 1 tablespoon chili powder
- 2 garlic cloves, minced
- 1 teaspoon chipotle chili pepper, chopped
- ½ teaspoon cumin, ground
- 16 ounces canned black beans, drained and rinsed
- 2 tablespoons cilantro, chopped
- 1 cup tomatoes, chopped

Directions:

1. Add red bell peppers, onion, dill, mushrooms, chili powder, garlic, chili pepper, cumin, black beans, and tomatoes to your Slow Cooker.
2. Stir well.
3. Place lid and cook on HIGH for 4 hours.
4. Sprinkle cilantro on top.
5. Serve and enjoy!

Nutrition:

- Calories: 211
- Fat: 3g
- Carbs: 22g
- Protein: 5g
- Sodium: 40mg

CHAPTER 12:

Dinner

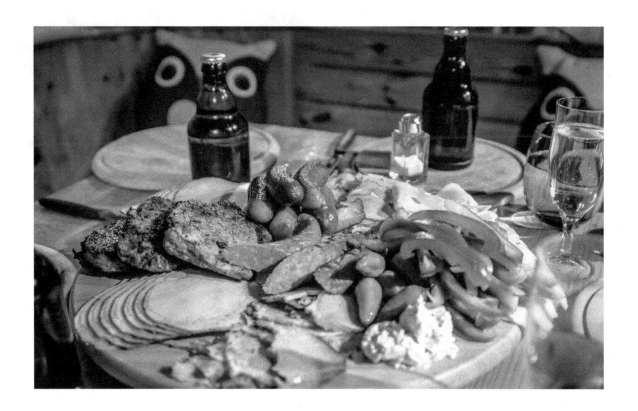

Hearty Chicken Liver Stew

- **Preparation time: 10 minutes**
- **Cooking time: 15 minutes**
- **Servings: 2**

Ingredients:

- 10 ounces chicken livers
- 1 onion, chopped
- 2 ounces sour cream
- 1 tablespoon olive oil
- Sunflower seeds to taste

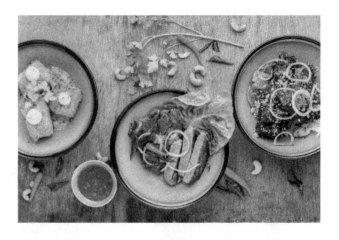

Directions:

1. Take a pan and place it over medium heat.
2. Add oil and let it heat up.
3. Add onions and fry until just browned.
4. Add livers and season with sunflower seeds.
5. Cook until livers are half cooked.
6. Transfer the mix to a stew pot.
7. Add sour cream and cook for 20 minutes.
8. Serve and enjoy!

Nutrition:

- Calories: 146
- Fat: 9g
- Carbs: 2g
- Protein: 15g
- Sodium: 350mg

Chicken and Carrot Stew

- **Preparation time: 15 minutes**
- **Cooking time: 6 minutes**
- **Servings: 2**

Ingredients:

- 4 boneless chicken breast, cubed
- 3 cups of carrots, peeled and cubed
- 1 cup onion, chopped
- 1 cup tomatoes, chopped
- 1 teaspoon of dried thyme
- 2 cups of chicken broth
- 2 garlic cloves, minced
- Sunflower seeds and pepper as needed

Directions:

1. Add all of the listed ingredients to a Slow Cooker.
2. Stir and close the lid.
3. Cook for 6 hours.
4. Serve hot and enjoy!

Nutrition:

- Calories: 182
- Fat: 3g
- Carbs: 10g
- Protein: 39g
- Sodium: 120mg

Bulgur Appetizer Salad

- **Preparation Time: 30 minutes**
- **Cooking time: 0 minutes**
- **Servings: 4**

Ingredients:

- 1 cup bulgur
- 2 cups hot water
- Black pepper to the taste
- 2 cups corn
- 1 cucumber, chopped
- 2 tablespoons lemon juice
- 2 tablespoons balsamic vinegar
- ¼ cup olive oil

Directions:

1. In a bowl, mix bulgur with the water, cover, leave aside for 30 minutes, fluff with a fork, and transfer to a salad bowl.
2. Add corn, cucumber, oil with lemon juice, vinegar, and pepper, toss, divide into small cups and serve.

Nutrition:

- Calories 130
- Fat: 2g
- Fiber: 2g
- Carbs: 7g
- Protein: 6g
- Sodium: 70mg

Greek Party Dip

- **Preparation Time: 10 minutes**
- **Cooking time: 0 minutes**
- **Servings: 4**

Ingredients:

- ½ cup coconut cream
- 1 cup fat-free Greek yogurt
- 2 teaspoons dill, dried
- 2 teaspoons thyme, dried
- 1 teaspoon sweet paprika
- 2 teaspoons no-salt-added sun-dried tomatoes, chopped
- 2 teaspoons parsley, chopped
- 2 teaspoons chives, chopped
- Black pepper to the taste

Directions:

1. In a bowl, mix cream with yogurt, dill with thyme, paprika, tomatoes, parsley, chives, and pepper, stir well, divide into smaller bowls and serve as a dip.

Nutrition:

- Calories 100
- Fat: 1g
- Fiber: 4g
- Carbs: 8g
- Protein: 3g
- Sodium: 75mg

Cheesy Mushrooms Caps

- **Preparation Time: 10 minutes**
- **Cooking time: 30 minutes**
- **Servings: 20**

Ingredients:

- 20 white mushroom caps
- 1 garlic clove, minced
- 3 tablespoons parsley, chopped
- 2 yellow onions, chopped
- Black pepper to the taste
- ½ cup low-fat parmesan, grated
- ¼ cup low-fat mozzarella, grated
- A drizzle of olive oil
- 2 tablespoons non-fat yogurt

Directions:

2. Heat up a pan with some oil over medium heat, add garlic and onion, stir, cook for 10 minutes and transfer to a bowl.
3. Add black pepper, garlic, parsley, mozzarella, parmesan, and yogurt, stir well, stuff the mushroom caps with this mix, arrange them on a lined baking sheet, bake in the oven at 400 degrees F for 20 minutes and serve them as an appetizer.

Nutrition:

- Calories: 100
- Fat: 1g
- Fiber: 4g
- Carbs: 8g
- Protein: 3g
- Sodium: 75mg

Mozzarella Cauliflower Bars

- **Preparation Time: 10 minutes**
- **Cooking time: 40 minutes**
- **Servings: 12**

Ingredients:

- 1 big cauliflower head, riced
- ½ cup low-fat mozzarella cheese, shredded
- ¼ cup egg whites
- 1 teaspoon Italian seasoning
- Black pepper to the taste

Directions:

1. Spread the cauliflower rice on a lined baking sheet, cook in the oven at 375 ° F for 20 minutes, transfer to a bowl, add black pepper, cheese, seasoning, and egg whites, stir well, spread into a rectangle pan, and press well on the bottom.
2. Introduce in the oven at 375 ° F, bake for 20 minutes, cut into 12 bars, and serve as a snack.

Nutrition:

- Calories 140
- Fat: 1g
- Fiber: 3g
- Carbs: 6g
- Protein: 6g
- Sodium: 110mg

Shrimp and Pineapple Salsa

- **Preparation Time: 10 minutes**
- **Cooking time: 40 minutes**
- **Servings: 4**

Ingredients:

- 1 pound large shrimp, peeled and deveined
- 20 ounces canned pineapple chunks
- 1 tablespoon garlic powder
- 1 cup red bell peppers, chopped
- Black pepper to the taste

Directions:

1. Place shrimp in a baking dish, add pineapple, garlic, bell peppers, and black pepper, toss a bit, introduce in the oven, bake at 375 ° F for 40 minutes.
2. Divide into small bowls and serve cold.

Nutrition:

- Calories 170
- Fat: 5g
- Fiber: 4g
- Carbs: 15g
- Sodium: 210mg
- Protein: 11g

Chicken Rolls with Pesto

- **Preparation Time: 20 minutes**
- **Cooking time: 30 minutes**
- **Servings: 1**

Ingredients:

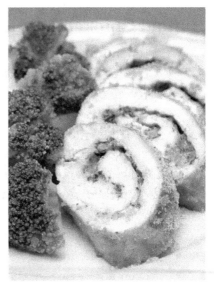

- Tablespoon pine nuts
- Yeast tablets
- Garlic cloves (chopped)
- Fresh basil
- Olive oil
- Chicken breast ready to slice:
- Preheat the oven to 175 ° C.
- Place the pine nuts in a dry pan and heat to a golden brown over medium heat for 3 minutes. Place on a plate and set aside.
- Place pine nuts, yeast flakes, and garlic in a food processor and grind finely.
- Add basil and oil and mix briefly until you get pesto.

Directions

1. Season with salt and pepper.
2. Place each piece of the chicken breast between 2 pieces of plastic wrap. 7 Roll in a frying pan or pasta until the chicken breasts grow out.
3. 0.6 cm thick.
4. Remove the plastic wrap, then apply pesto to the chicken.
5. Roll up the chicken breast and tie it with the cocktail skewers.
6. Season with salt and pepper.
7. Dissolve the coconut oil in the pan and use a high temperature to brown all sides of the chicken skin.
8. Place the chicken rolls on a baking sheet, place in the oven, and bake for 15 to 20 minutes, until cooked.
9. Slice it diagonally and serve it with other pesto sauce.
10. It was served with tomato salad.

Nutrition:

- Calories: 150
- Sodium: 33mg
- Fat: 4.3g
- Carbs: 15.4g
- Protein: 1.6g

Buffalo Chicken Lettuce Wraps

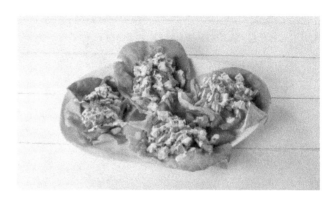

- **Preparation time: 35 minutes**
- **Cooking time: 10 minutes**
- **Servings: 2**

Ingredients:

- 3 chicken breasts, boneless and cubed
- 20 slices of almond butter lettuce leaves
- ¾ cup cherry tomatoes halved
- 1 avocado, chopped
- ¼ cup green onions, diced
- ½ cup ranch dressing
- ¾ cup hot sauce

Directions:

1. Take a mixing bowl and add chicken cubes and hot sauce, mix.
2. Place in the fridge and let it marinate for 30 minutes.
3. Preheat your oven to 400 degrees F.
4. Place coated chicken on a cookie pan and bake for 9 minutes.
5. Assemble lettuce serving cups with equal amounts of lettuce, green onions, tomatoes, ranch dressing, and cubed chicken.
6. Serve and enjoy!

Nutrition:

- Calories: 106
- Fat: 6g
- Carbs: 2g
- Protein: 5g
- Sodium 120mg

Sweet and sour sauce

- **Preparation Time: 10 minutes**
- **Cooking time: 10 minutes**
- **Servings: 1**

Ingredients

- Apple cider vinegar
- 1/2 tablespoon tomato paste
- A teaspoon of coconut amino acid
- Bamboo spoon
- Water treatment
- Chopped vegetables.

Directions

1. Mix kudzu powder with five tablespoons of cold water to make a paste.
2. Then put all the other spices in the pot, then add the kudzu paste.
3. Melt coconut oil in a pan and fry onions.
4. Add green pepper, cabbage, cabbage, and bean sprouts, then cook until the vegetables are tender.
5. Add pineapple and cashew nuts and mix a few times.
6. Just pour a little spice into the pot.

Nutrition:

- Calories: 3495
- Sodium: 33mg
- Fat: 4.5g
- Carbs: 16.5g
- Protein: 1.7g

Coconut Curry Cauliflower Soup

- **Preparation Time:** 10 minutes
- **Cooking Time:** 25 minutes
- **Servings:** 10

Ingredients:

- 2 tablespoons olive oil
- 1 onion, chopped
- 3 tablespoons yellow curry paste
- 2 heads cauliflower, sliced into florets
- 32 oz. vegetable broth
- 1 cup coconut milk
- Minced fresh cilantro

Directions:

1. In a pan over medium heat, add the oil.
2. Cook onion for 3 minutes.
3. Stir in the curry paste and cook for 2 minutes.
4. Add the cauliflower florets.
5. Pour in the broth.
6. Increase the heat to high and bring to a boil.
7. Lower the heat to medium.
8. Cook while covered for 20 minutes.
9. Add the coconut milk and cook for an additional minute.
10. Puree in a blender.
11. Garnish with fresh cilantro.

Nutrition:

- Calories: 138
- Fat: 11.8g
- Sodium: 430mg
- Carbs: 6.4g
- Fiber: 3g
- Protein: 3.6g

Mexican Soup

- **Preparation Time:** 5 minutes
- **Cooking Time:** 15 minutes
- **Servings:** 4

Ingredients:

- 2 teaspoons olive oil
- 1 lb. chicken thighs (skinless and boneless), sliced into smaller pieces
- 1 tablespoon taco seasoning
- 1 cup frozen corn
- 1 cup salsa
- 32 oz. chicken broth

Directions:

1. In a pan over medium heat, add oil.
2. Cook chicken for 7 minutes, stirring frequently.
3. Add the taco seasoning and mix well.
4. Add the rest of the ingredients.
5. Bring to a boil.
6. Reduce heat to low and simmer for 5 minutes.
7. Remove fat before serving.

Nutrition:

- Calories: 322
- Fat: 12.6g
- Sodium: 1214mg
- Carbs: 12.2g
- Fiber: 2.1g
- Protein: 39.6g

Roasted Tomato Soup

- **Preparation Time:** 20 minutes
- **Cooking Time:** 25 minutes
- **Servings:** 6

Ingredients:

- Cooking spray
- 3 ½ lb. tomatoes, sliced into half
- 1 onion, sliced into wedges
- 2 cloves garlic, sliced in half
- 2 tablespoons olive oil
- Salt and pepper to taste
- 2 tablespoons fresh thyme leaves
- 12 fresh basil leaves

Directions:

1. Preheat your oven to 400 degrees F.
2. Put the onion, garlic and tomatoes on a baking pan coated with cooking spray.
3. Drizzle vegetables with olive oil and toss.
4. Season with salt, pepper and thyme.
5. Roast for 30 minutes.
6. Place the tomato mixture and basil leaves in a blender.
7. Pulse until smooth.

Nutrition:

- Calories: 99
- Fat: 5.3g
- Sodium: 14mg
- Carbs: 13g
- Fiber: 4g
- Protein: 2.7g

Squash Soup

- **Preparation Time: 15 minutes**
- **Cooking Time: 20 minutes**
- **Servings: 6**

Ingredients:

- 5 leeks, sliced
- 2 tablespoons butter
- 4 cups chicken broth
- ¼ teaspoon dried thyme
- 4 cups butternut squash, peeled and cubed
- ¼ teaspoon pepper
- 2 cups cheddar cheese, shredded
- 1 green onion, thinly sliced
- ¼ cup sour cream

Directions:

1. In a pan over medium heat, sauté the leeks in butter.
2. Add the broth, thyme, squash and pepper.
3. Bring to a boil and then simmer for 15 minutes.
4. Let it cool.
5. Transfer the mixture to a blender.
6. Pulse until smooth.
7. Stir in the cheese.
8. Garnish with the green onion and sour cream before serving.

Nutrition:

- Calories: 320
- Fat: 19.6g
- Sodium: 794mg
- Carbs: 23.2g
- Fiber: 3.3g
- Protein: 15.1g

Vegetable Soup

- **Preparation Time: 5 minutes**
- **Cooking Time: 30 minutes**
- **Servings: 6**

Ingredients:

- 2 tablespoons olive oil
- 1 onion, diced
- 2 bell peppers, diced
- 2 cloves garlic, minced
- 2 cups green beans, sliced
- 1 head cauliflower, sliced into florets
- 1 tablespoon Italian seasoning
- 8 cups chicken broth
- 30 oz. diced tomatoes
- Salt and pepper to taste
- 2 dried bay leaves

Directions:

1. Pour the olive oil into a pot over medium heat.
2. Sauté the onion and bell peppers for 7 minutes.
3. Add the garlic and cook for 1 minute.
4. Add the rest of the ingredients.
5. Bring to a boil.
6. Reduce to medium-low.
7. Simmer for 20 minutes.

Nutrition:

- Calories: 168
- Fat: 7.7g
- Sodium: 1043mg
- Carbs: 17.1g
- Fiber: 5.1g
- Protein: 9.9g

Mashed Cauliflower with Chives

- **Preparation Time:** 15 minutes
- **Cooking Time:** 25 minutes
- **Servings:** 4

Ingredients:

- 2 cups chicken broth
- 2 heads cauliflower, cored and sliced into florets
- ¼ cup fresh chives, chopped
- ¼ cup Parmesan cheese, grated
- Salt and pepper to taste

Directions:

1. In a pot over medium heat, pour in the chicken broth.
2. Add the cauliflower.
3. Bring to a boil and then simmer for 20 minutes.
4. Transfer cauliflower to a blender.
5. Pulse until smooth.
6. Stir in the chives and cheese.
7. Season with salt and pepper.

Nutrition:

- Calories: 98
- Fat: 3.8g
- Sodium: 551mg
- Carbs: 8.1g
- Fiber: 3.4g
- Protein: 9.6g

Garlic Parmesan Zucchini

- **Preparation Time: 5 minutes**
- **Cooking Time: 20 minutes**
- **Servings: 6**

Ingredients:

- ¼ cup Parmesan cheese
- ¼ cup mayonnaise
- 1 clove garlic, minced
- Salt to taste
- 2 zucchinis, sliced

Directions:

1. Preheat your oven to 400 ° F.
2. Combine all the ingredients except the zucchini.
3. Spread mixture on top of zucchini.
4. Bake in the oven for 20 minutes.

Nutrition:

- Calories: 79
- Fat: 5.4g
- Sodium: 190mg
- Carbs: 5g
- Fiber: 0.7g
- Protein: 3.9g

Cheesy Roasted Broccoli

- **Preparation Time: 5 minutes**
- **Cooking Time: 10 minutes**
- **Servings: 6**

Ingredients:

- ¼ cup ranch dressing
- 4 cups broccoli florets
- ¼ cup heavy whipping cream
- ½ cup cheddar cheese, shredded
- Salt and pepper to taste

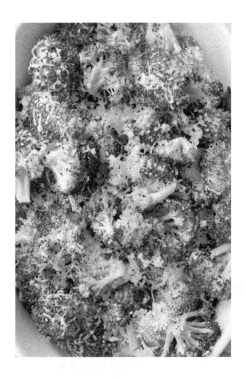

Directions:

1. Preheat your oven to 375 degrees F.
2. Put all the ingredients in a bowl and mix.
3. Arrange the broccoli mix on a baking dish.
4. Bake in the oven for 10 minutes or until tender enough.

Nutrition:

- Calories: 79
- Fat: 5.2g
- Sodium: 137mg
- Carbs: 4.8g
- Fiber: 1.6g
- Protein: 4.3g

Stir Fried Green Beans

- **Preparation Time:** 20 minutes
- **Cooking Time:** 10 minutes
- **Servings:** 4

Ingredients:

- 1 lb. green beans, trimmed and sliced
- 2 tablespoons peanut oil
- 2 tablespoons garlic, chopped
- ½ onion, sliced
- Salt to taste
- 1 tablespoon water
- 2 tablespoons oyster sauce

Directions:

1. Add peanut oil to a pan over high heat.
2. Heat it for 2 minutes.
3. Add the garlic and onion.
4. Cook for 30 seconds.
5. Add the beans and season with salt.
6. Cook for 2 minutes.
7. Pour in the water and cover the pan.
8. Steam for 5 minutes.
9. Stir in the oyster sauce and cook for 2 minutes.

Nutrition:

- Calories: 108
- Fat: 1.2g
- Sodium: 102mg
- Carbs: 11g
- Fiber: 4.3g
- Protein: 2.5g

Roasted Asparagus

- **Preparation Time: 10 minutes**
- **Cooking Time: 20 minutes**
- **Servings: 4**

Ingredients:

- 1 lb. asparagus
- 1 tablespoon peanut oil
- 1 teaspoon coconut oil
- 1 tablespoon soy sauce
- 1 teaspoon sesame oil
- 2 teaspoons sesame seeds

Directions:

1. Preheat your oven to 400 degrees F.
2. Arrange the asparagus spears on a baking pan.
3. Brush with peanut oil.
4. Roast for 15 minutes.
5. While waiting, mix the coconut oil, soy sauce, and sesame oil.
6. Brush the asparagus with the mixture and roast for 7 minutes.
7. Sprinkle with sesame seeds before serving.

Nutrition:

- Calories: 83
- Fat: 6.5g
- Sodium: 228mg
- Carbs: 5.1g
- Fiber: 2.6g
- Protein: 3g

CHAPTER 13:

Snacks and Dessert

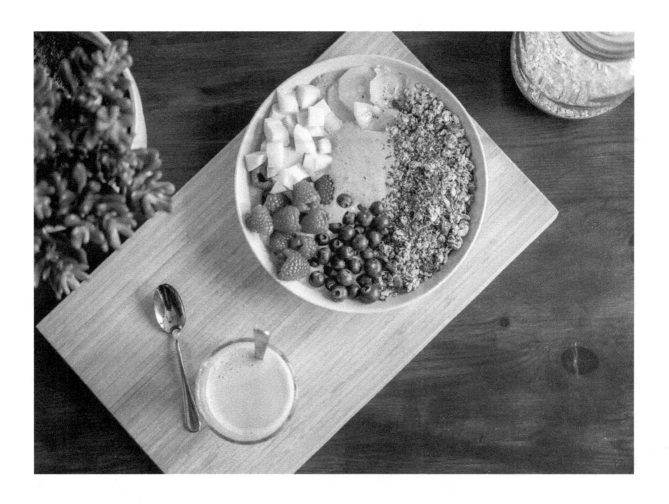

Cocoa Bars

- **Preparation Time: 2 hours**
- **Cooking time: 0 minutes**
- **Servings: 12**

Ingredients:

- 1 cup unsweetened cocoa chips
- 2 cups rolled oats
- 1 cup low-fat peanut butter
- ½ cup chia seeds
- ½ cup raisins
- ¼ cup coconut sugar
- ½ cup coconut milk

Directions:

1. Put one and ½ cups oats in your blender, pulse well, transfer this to a bowl, add the rest of the oats, cocoa chips, chia seeds, raisins, sugar, and milk,
2. Stir well, spread this into a square pan, press well, keep in the fridge for 2 hours, slice into 12 bars and serve.

Nutrition:

- Calories: 198
- Fat: 5g
- Fiber: 4g
- Carbs: 10g
- Protein: 89g
- Sodium: 70mg

Apple and Pecans Bowls

- **Preparation Time: 10 minutes**
- **Cooking time: 0 minutes**
- **Servings: 4**

Ingredients:

- 4 big apples, cored, peeled and cubed
- 2 teaspoons lemon juice
- ¼ cup pecans, chopped

Directions:

1. In a bowl, mix apples with lemon juice and pecans, toss, divide into small bowls, and serve as a snack.

Nutrition:

- Calories: 120
- Fat: 4g
- Fiber: 3g
- Carbs: 12g
- Protein: 3g
- Sodium: 70mg

Shrimp Muffins

- **Preparation Time: 10 minutes**
- **Cooking time: 45 minutes**
- **Servings: 6**

Ingredients:

- 1 spaghetti squash, peeled and halved
- 2 tablespoons avocado mayonnaise
- 1 cup low-fat mozzarella cheese, shredded
- 8 ounces' shrimp, peeled, cooked, and chopped
- 1 and ½ cups almond flour
- 1 teaspoon parsley, dried
- 1 garlic clove, minced
- Black pepper to the taste
- Cooking spray

Directions:

1. Arrange the squash on a lined baking sheet, introduce in the oven at 375 ° F, bake for 30 minutes, scrape flesh into a bowl.
2. Add pepper, parsley flakes, flour, shrimp, mayo, and mozzarella and stir well, divide this mix into a muffin tray greased with cooking spray
3. Bake in the oven at 375 degrees F for 15 minutes and serve them cold as a snack.

Nutrition:

- Calories: 140
- Fat: 2g
- Fiber: 4g
- Carbs: 14g
- Protein: 12g
- Sodium: 50mg

Vanilla Biscuits

- **Preparation Time: 15 minutes**
- **Cooking Time: 40 minutes**
- **Serving: 1**

Ingredients:

- 5 eggs
- ½ cup coconut flour
- ½ cup wheat flour
- 1/3 cup Erythritol
- 1 teaspoon vanilla extract
- Cooking spray

Directions:

1. Crack the eggs in the mixing bowl and mix it up with the help of the hand mixer.

2. Add Erythritol and keep mixing the egg mixture until it will be changed into the lemon color.

3. Add wheat flour, coconut flour, and vanilla extract.

4. Mix it for 30 seconds.

5. Spray the baking tray with cooking spray.

6. Pour the biscuit mixture in the tray and flatten it.

7. Bake it for 40 minutes at 350^0 F.

8. When the biscuit is cooked, cut it into squares and serve.

Nutrition:

- Calories 132
- Fat 4.7g
- Fiber 4.3g
- Carbs 28.3g
- Protein 7g
- Sodium: 20mg

Cinnamon Apple Chips

- **Preparation Time: 10 minutes**
- **Cooking time: 2 hours**
- **Servings: 4**

Ingredients:

- Cooking spray
- 2 teaspoons cinnamon powder
- 2 apples, cored and thinly sliced

Directions:

1. Arrange apple slices on a lined baking sheet, spray them with cooking oil, sprinkle cinnamon, introduce them in the oven, and bake at 300 ° F for 2 hours.
2. Divide into bowls and serve as a snack.

Nutrition:

- Calories: 80
- Fat: 0g
- Fiber: 3g
- Carbs: 7g
- Protein: 4g
- Sodium: 70mg

Coconut-Mint Bars

Preparation Time: 35 minutes

Cooking Time: 1 minute

Serving: 1

Ingredients:

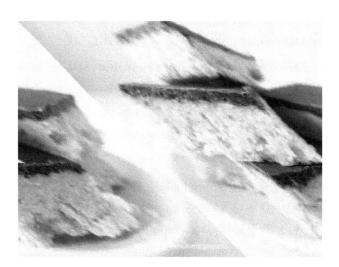

- 3 tablespoons coconut butter
- ½ cup coconut flakes
- 1 egg, beaten
- 1 tablespoon cocoa powder
- 3 oz graham crackers, crushed
- 2 tablespoons Erythritol
- 3 tablespoons butter
- 1 teaspoon mint extract
- 1 teaspoon stevia powder
- 1 teaspoon of cocoa powder
- 1 tablespoon almond butter, melted

Directions:

1. Churn together coconut butter, coconut flakes, and 1 tablespoon of cocoa powder.
2. Microwave the mixture for 1 minute or until it is melted.
3. Chill the liquid for 1 minute and fast add egg. Whisk it until homogenous and smooth.
4. Add and stir the liquid in the crushed graham crackers and transfer the mixture to the mold. Flatten it well with the help of the spoon.
5. After this, blend Erythritol, butter, mint extract, and stevia powder.
6. When the mixture is fluffy; place it over the graham crackers layer.
7. Mix 1 teaspoon of cocoa powder and almond butter.
8. Sprinkle the cocoa liquid on the cooked mixture and flatten it.
9. Refrigerate the dessert for 30 minutes.
10. .cut it into the bars.

Nutrition:

- Calories 213
- Fat 16.3g
- Fiber 2.9g
- Carbs 20g
- Protein 3.5g
- Sodium: 10mg

Strawberry & Nut Granola

- **Preparation Time: 10 minutes**
- **Cooking time: 50 minutes**
- **Servings: 12**

Ingredients:

- 200g (7oz) oats
- 250g (9oz) buckwheat flakes
- 100g (3½ oz.) walnuts, chopped
- 100g (3½ oz.) almonds, chopped
- 100g (3½ oz.) dried strawberries
- 1½ teaspoons ground ginger
- 1½ teaspoons ground cinnamon
- 120mls (4fl oz.) olive oil
- 2 tablespoon honey

Directions:

1. Combine the oats, buckwheat flakes, nuts, ginger, and cinnamon. In a saucepan, warm the oil and honey. Stir until the honey has melted.
2. Pour the warm oil into the dry ingredients and mix well. Spread the mixture out on a large baking tray (or two) and bake in the oven at 150°C (300F) for around 50 minutes until the granola is golden.
3. Allow it to cool. Add in the dried berries. Store in an airtight container until ready to use.
4. Can be served with yogurt, milk, or even dry as a handy snack.

Nutrition:

- Calories: 391
- Fat: 0g
- Fiber: 6g
- Sodium: 70mg
- Carbs: 3g
- Protein: 8g

Chilled Strawberry & Walnut Porridge

- **Preparation Time: 10 minutes**
- **Cooking time: 0 minutes**
- **Servings: 1**

Ingredients:

- 100g (3½ oz.) strawberries
- 50g (2oz) rolled oats
- 4 walnut halves, chopped
- 1 teaspoon chia seeds
- 200mls (7fl oz.) unsweetened soya milk
- 100ml (3½ FL oz.) water

Directions:

1. Place the strawberries, oats, soya milk, and water into a blender and process until smooth.
2. Stir in the chia seeds and mix well.
3. Chill in the fridge overnight and serve in the morning with a sprinkling of chopped walnuts.
4. It's simple and delicious.

Nutrition:

- Calories 384
- Fat: 2g
- Sodium: 60mg
- Fiber: 5g
- Carbs: 3g
- Protein: 7g

Fruit & Nut Yogurt Crunch

- **Preparation Time: 5 minutes**
- **Cooking time: 0 minutes**
- **Servings: 1**

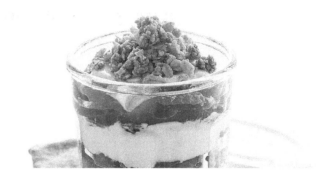

Ingredients:

1. 100g (3½ oz.) plain Greek yogurt
2. 50g (2oz) strawberries, chopped
3. 6 walnut halves, chopped
4. Sprinkling of cocoa powder

Directions:

1. Stir half of the chopped strawberries into the yogurt.
2. Using a glass, place a layer of yogurt with a sprinkling of strawberries and walnuts, followed by another layer of the same until you reach the top of the glass.
3. Garnish with walnuts pieces and a dusting of cocoa powder.

Nutrition:

- Calories: 296
- Fat: 4g
- Fiber: 2g
- Carbs: 5g
- Protein: 9g
- Sodium: 70mg

Chicken Quesadilla

- **Preparation time: 10 minutes**
- **Cooking time: 35 minutes**
- **Servings: 2**

Ingredients:

- ¼ cup ranch dressing
- ½ cup cheddar cheese, shredded
- 20 slices bacon, center-cut
- 2 cups grilled chicken, sliced

Directions:

1. Re-heat your oven to 400 ° F.
2. Line baking sheet using parchment paper.
3. Weave bacon into two rectangles and bake for 30 minutes.
4. Lay grilled chicken over bacon square, drizzling ranch dressing on top.
5. Sprinkle cheddar cheese and top with another bacon square.
6. Bake for 5 minutes more.
7. Slice and serve.
8. Enjoy!

Nutrition

- Calories: 619
- Fat: 35g
- Carbs: 2g
- Protein: 79g
- Sodium: 250mg

Spicy Pumpkin Seeds Bowls

- **Preparation Time: 10 minutes**
- **Cooking time: 20 minutes**
- **Servings: 6**

Ingredients:

- ½ tablespoon chili powder
- ½ teaspoon cayenne pepper
- 2 cups pumpkin seeds
- 2 teaspoons lime juice

Directions:

1. Spread pumpkin seeds on a lined baking sheet, add lime juice, cayenne, and chili powder, toss well, introduce in the oven, roast at 275 ° F for 20 minutes.
2. Divide into small bowls and serve as a snack.

Nutrition:

- Calories: 170
- Fat: 2g
- Fiber: 7g
- Carbs: 12g
- Protein: 6g
- Sodium: 70mg

CHAPTER 14:

Measurement Conversion Table

Liquid Measures			
1 cup	8 fluid ounces	1/2 pint	237 ml
2 cups	16 fluid ounces	1 pint	474 ml
4 cups	32 fluid ounces	1 quart	946 ml
2 pints	32 fluid ounces	1 quart	946 ml
4 quarts	128 fluid ounces	1 gallon	3.784 liters

Dry Measures				
3 teaspoons	1 tablespoon	1/2 ounce	14.3 grams	
2 tablespoons	1/8 cup	1 fluid ounce	28.3 grams	
4 tablspoons	1/4 cup	2 fluid ounces	56.7 grams	
5 1/3 tablespoons	1/3 cup	2.6 fluid ounces	75.6 grams	
8 tablespoons	1/2 cup	4 ounces	113.4 grams	1 stick butter
12 tablespoons	3/4 cup	6 ounces	.375 pound	170 grams
32 tablespoons	2 cups	16 ounces	1 pound	453.6 grams
64 tablespoons	4 cups	32 ounces	2 pounds	907 grams

Conclusion

If you are reading this book, then you have already taken an important step by making your health, or the health of a loved one, a priority—congratulations! One of the biggest parts of becoming healthy is taking control and becoming informed. This book will make it easy for you to embrace a diet proven to lower blood pressure, cholesterol, and the risk for a number of chronic diseases. And you can start all this right now. Change your thinking about dieting, evolve from limiting yourself to thinking about what you can add to your diet and what you can add to your life. Find your inner motivation, whether it is to be able to keep up with your grandchildren or to finally walk that half-marathon—harness your inner drive and make the commitment to optimize your health. If you stick with it and believe in yourself, you're going to reach your goal. Get ready to embrace the new you. I believe in you.

Remember the Dash is designed not for losing weight but to lower blood pressure. It does this by balancing your mineral intake. Sodium promotes fluid retention and raises blood pressure, but other minerals like potassium and magnesium have the opposite effect. You do need salt, of course, but since most Americans consume far too much sodium, the balance between all these important minerals is disrupted, leading to high blood pressure. The Dash diet addresses this issue.

The Dash diet also includes a simplified system based on numbers of portions per day, rather than counting calories, which makes it easy to follow.

High blood pressure and diabetes are not comparable to having a cold, which is mostly of a short-term nature. They are not symptoms that regulate themselves again, but rather warning signals from the body — red alert! So don't take it lightly!

The fatal thing about high blood pressure is that the symptoms are often inconspicuous and unspecific, such as headache, dizziness, nosebleeds, chest pressure, and may even be absent completely. So it happens that many people who have high blood pressure do not know anything about it.

The symptoms of diabetes are also very insidious, such as tiredness and a decline in performance, leg cramps, severe thirst, and cravings.

Therefore, have your blood pressure and blood sugar levels checked regularly and change your diet. It is not wise to wait until a critical moment is reached, and the emergency doctor needs to be called. And then taking medication is not the solution to the problem.

The diet presented here is a diet that does not require any major restrictions in life: just more of the healthy and less of the unhealthy. With a few tricks it is not difficult to make your diet tasty and tasty without losing the quality of life.

Combine it with regular exercise and healthy sport, and you are on the right side.

I hope that I could convey to you how important a healthy diet is in our lives and how the Dash diet can support you.

If you enjoyed this book, I want to ask you a favor. Would you be so kind as to leave a review for this book? I would be very grateful because you support my work with it.

I wish you good luck, happiness, and health on your path in life!

Recipe Index

Sheila J. Baker

DASH DIET COOKBOOK

Easy and Healthy Recipes with Specific Nutritional Values.
Change Your Eating Habits to Lower Your Blood Pressure and Lose
Weight with Low Sodium Meals

Introduction of Dash Diet Cookbook

Generally speaking, most people who are looking to start the DASH diet are people who suffer from high blood pressure themselves or have a family member that does.

Men are more likely to have hypertension issues, especially after the age of 45, and a significant amount of patients with diabetes will experience these symptoms as well. Also, put at risk are individuals who are overweight. However, hypertension can happen to anyone.

DASH is an acronym for Dietary Approaches to Stop Hypertension. The diet is centered on eating a balanced combination of lean meats, vegetables, whole grains, and fruits, and keeping sodium intake between two-thirds and one tablespoon of salt per day depending on the reasons for starting the diet and the results you are seeking.

The DASH diet also focuses on keeping fats, added sugars, and red meat to a lower level. As with all diets, there is a happy medium for keeping true to the diet.

When you experience the symptoms of hypertension for extended amounts of time, you are more at risk for heart disease, kidney issues, and higher glucose levels leading to diabetes. You also are at a higher risk of early mortality.

However, following the simple to understand guidelines of the DASH Diet will help to bring your blood pressure numbers to a more manageable level and help you to be healthier in the long run, bringing your chances of living a much more fulfilling life for you.

When you work towards your goals on the DASH Diet, you will start to see the results rather quickly which will help you to keep your willpower working towards your personal goals.

CHAPTER 15:

Understanding the Dash Diet

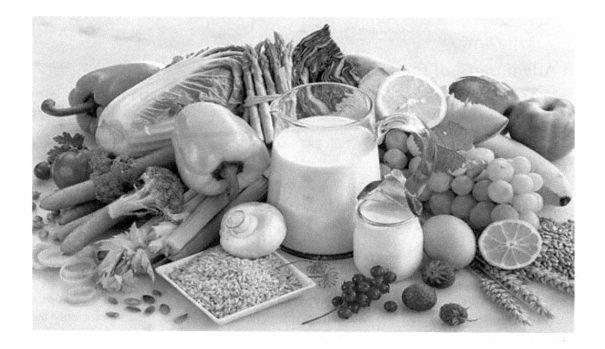

Dietary Approaches to Stop Hypertension is one of the most effective organic treatments of all health problems related to high blood pressure or fluid build-up in the body. These approaches come with a complete program, which places emphasis on the diet as well as lifestyle changes. Commonly called the DASH diet, the major target is to reduce the sodium content of your diet by omitting table salt directly or reducing the intake through other ingredients. There are two minerals that work against each other to maintain the body fluid balance: those are sodium and potassium. In perfect proportions, these two control the release and retention of fluids in the body. In the case of environmental or genetic complexities or a high sodium diet, the balance is disturbed so much that it puts our heart at risk by elevating systolic and diastolic blood pressures.

Origin of the DASH Diet

This dietary plan came to the knowledge of nutritionists after several research studies were conducted to treat hypertension focused on diet in order to avoid medication's side effects. It was seen as a way to reduce the blood pressure using healthy, nourishing food and following an active routine. The main goal was to cure hypertension, so it was soon termed as the Dietary Approaches to Stop Hypertension (DASH).

However, its broad-scale effects showed greater efficiency than just reducing hypertension, and people started using it to treat obesity, diabetes, cancer, and cardiac disorders.

To study the impact of sodium intake, a scientist used three experimental groups. Each group was assigned a diet with varying sodium levels. One was to take 3300 mg sodium per day; the second had to use 2300 mg per day, and the third one was put on a diet having 1500 mg sodium per day, about two-thirds of a teaspoon of salt. By restricting the sodium content, all participants showed decreased blood pressure. But the group with the least amount of sodium intake showed the most alleviation in the blood pressure levels. Thus, it was identified that 1500 mg of sodium per day is the threshold amount to maintain blood pressure.

Health Advantages of the DASH Diet

Besides hypertension, there are several health advantages that later came to light as experts recorded the conditions people experience after choosing the diet. Here are some of the known benefits of the DASH diet:

Alleviated Blood Pressure

It is the most obvious and direct outcome of this dietary routine as it restricts the sodium intake, which rightly reduces the risks of high blood pressure by keeping the blood consistency to near normal. People with hypertension disorder should restrict sodium intake the most, whereas others should keep the intake as per the described limits, 1500 mg per day.

Maintained Cholesterol Levels

Since a DASH diet promotes greater use of vegetables, fruits, whole grains, beans, and nuts, it can provide enough fiber to regulate our metabolism and digestive functions. Moreover, it promotes only lean meats and no saturated fats, which also helps to maintain cholesterol levels in the body. Such fats have to be replaced with healthy cholesterol fats to keep the heart running.

Weight Maintenance

Weight loss is another primary objective for people on the DASH diet. With a nutritious and clean diet, anyone can lose their excess weight. Moreover, the DASH diet also promotes proper physical exercise every day, which also proves to be significant in reducing obesity. Sometimes, obesity is the result of inflammation or fluid imbalances in the body, and the DASH diet can even cure that through its progressive health approach.

Reduced Risks of Osteoporosis

Osteoporosis is the degeneration of the bones, and there are many factors associated with it; at the base of it is the decrease of calcium and vitamin D in the body. The DASH diet provides ways and meals to fill this deficiency gap and reduce the risks of osteoporosis, especially in women.

Healthier Kidneys

Kidneys are what control the fluid balance of the body with the help of hormones and minerals. So, a smart diet that is designed with the sole purpose of aiding kidney functions can keep them healthy and functioning properly. Excess salt or oxalate intake can cause kidney stones. The DASH diet reduces the chances of these stones from building up in the kidneys.

Protection From Cancer

The DASH diet has been proven effective in preventing people from different types of cancer, like kidney, lung, prostate, esophagus, rectum, and colon cancers. The diet co-joins all the important factors which can fight against cancer and help prevent the development of cancerous cells.

Prevention From Diabetes

The DASH diet is effective in reducing insulin resistance, which is one of the common causes of diabetes in many people. Reduced weight, an active metabolism, maintained body fluids, daily exercises, increased water consumption, a low sodium diet, and a healthy gut or digestive system are all the factors that link the DASH diet with the reduced risks of diabetes in a person.

Improved Mental Health

Mental health is largely dependent on the type of food you eat. Anxiety, depression, and insomnia are all the outcomes of poor health and a bad lifestyle. The entire neural transmission is controlled by the electrolyte balance in the nervous system. With the DASH diet, you can create optimum conditions for efficient brain functions.

Less Risk of Heart Disease

Since the DASH diet is designed to control the varying blood pressure, it saves the heart from the negative impact of high blood pressure and prevents it from different diseases. Constant high blood pressure burdens the heart and causes the weakening of its walls and valves. Such risks are reduced with the help of the DASH diet.

The DASH Dietary Program

It's not just the sodium on which the DASH diet focuses; there are various forms and types of food that it limits. It also places a large emphasis on a certain amount of food per serving. It creates a special place or a box of food for the entire day and limits your daily intake to a value that would maintain a balance in the diet. Such control is hard to attain when you are not following the DASH diet, as the diet prescribes the entire roadmap to better dietary solutions. It is designed to change the ways we see our food and the way we consume it. It mainly works in two ways. First, it controls the quality of the meal, and second, it controls the quantity of the meal. By doing this, you can achieve increased health benefits that no other diet could guarantee. The food is first placed into categories, like fruits, vegetables, whole grains, beans, nuts, meat, or dairy, then you consider the health impact of each category; their share in a single meal or serving is suggested.

Research-Based Benefits of DASH Dieting

The National Institute of Health in the United States carried out early research on the significance of the DASH Diet. Scientists knew the impact of such a diet, but they needed proof to strengthen their claim. So, three different dietary plans were designed to check the impact. The plan with the most fruits, vegetables, beans, and no fat dairy items came out as the most effective in decreasing the diastolic and systolic blood pressures by 3 mmHg and 6 mmHg, respectively. While the DASH diet sets a limitation on certain food items, it also directs a person to controlled caloric intake. It keeps the daily caloric intake between 1600 to 3100. This fact becomes more relevant when there is obesity that has to be dealt with. By passing the Optimal Macronutrient Intake Trial for heart health, the DASH diet set the record of successfully reducing the routine fat intake, preventing all sorts of heart diseases.

It's a Long-Term Solution

Hypertension sufferers cannot always count on medications for long term health stability. No matter how effective the medicines are, they are not free from side effects. A change in diet and lifestyle can give long term treatment along with necessary prevention. Hypertension is not a temporary disorder; once a person has it, they are forever bound by this problem. It is not a matter of days, it's a matter of the rest of their life. That is why only dietary treatment can save the body from high blood pressure and the problems associated with it.

Helps Manage Type 2 Diabetes

To understand the relevance between the DASH diet and diabetes, it is important to look into the root causes of Type 2 Diabetes. High caloric food or increased body weight both make the body resistant to insulin. When you cross off both those factors, it becomes easier to control Type 2 Diabetes. The DASH diet works to manage both these factors. Firstly, through its regulated serving technique and secondly, through reducing obesity. It makes the body more sensitive to insulin; thus, it decreases the possible risks of high blood sugar levels. Moreover, with the dietary balance the DASH diet creates, it sets the bar for carbohydrate consumption, and in the absence of excess carbohydrates, the body can regulate its insulin production and its functions.

Ten Reasons Why the DASH Diet Truly Works

Talking about the DASH diet outside the theory and more in practice reveals more of its efficiency as a diet. Besides excess research and experiments, the true reasons for people looking into this diet are its certain features. It gives the feeling of ease and convenience, which makes the users more comfortable with its rules and regulations. Here are some of the reasons why the DASH

Diet works amazingly:

Easy to Adopt

The broad range of options available under the label of DASH diet makes it more flexible for all. This is the reason that people find it easier to switch to and harness its true health benefits. It makes adaptability easier for its users.

Promotes Exercise

It is most effective than all the other factors because not only does it focus on the food and its intake, but it also duly stresses daily exercises and routine physical activities. This is the reason why it produces quick, visible results.

All Inclusive

With few limitations, this Diet has taken every food item into its fold with certain modifications. It rightly guides us about the Dos and Don'ts of all the ingredients and prevents us from consuming those which are harmful to the body and its health.

A Well Balanced Approach

One of its biggest advantages is that it maintains balance in our diet, in our routine, our caloric intake, and our nutrition.

Good Caloric Check

Every meal we plan on the DASH diet is pre-calculated in terms of calories. We can easily keep track of the daily caloric intake and consequently restrict them easily by cutting off certain food items.

Prohibits Bad Food

The DASH diet suggests the use of more organic and fresh food and discourages the use of processed food and junk items available in stores. So, it creates better eating habits for the users.

Focused on Prevention

Though it is proven to be a cure for many diseases, it is described as more of a preventive strategy.

Slow Yet Progressive Changes

The diet is not highly restrictive and accommodates gradual changes towards achieving the ultimate health goal. You can set up your daily, weekly, or even monthly goals at your own convenience.

Long Term Effects

The results of the DASH diet are not just incredible, but they are also long-lasting. It is considered slow in progress, but the effects last longer.

Accelerates Metabolism

With its healthy approach to life, the DASH diet has the ability to activate our metabolism and boost it for better functioning of the body.

CHAPTER 16:

Breakfast & Smoothies

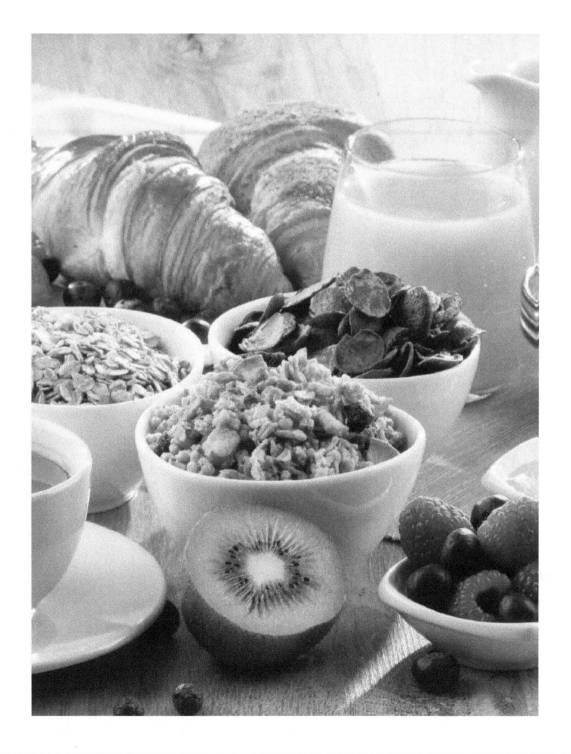

Yogurt & Banana Muffins

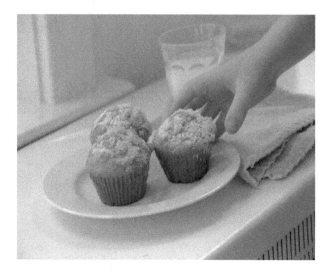

Preparation Time: 15 minutes

Cooking Time: 25 minutes

Servings: 2

Ingredients:

- 3 bananas, large & mashed
- 1 teaspoon baking soda
- 1 cup old fashioned rolled oats
- 2 tablespoons flaxseed, ground
- 1 cup whole wheat flour
- ¼ cup applesauce, unsweetened
- ½ cup plain yogurt
- ¼ cup brown sugar
- 2 teaspoons vanilla extract, pure

Directions:

1. Start by turning the oven to 355, and then get out a muffin tray. Grease it and then get out a bowl.
2. Mix your flaxseed, oats, soda, and flour in a bowl.
3. Mash your banana and then mix in your sugar, vanilla, yogurt, and applesauce. Stir in your oats mixture, making sure it's well combined. It's okay for it to be lumpy.
4. Divide between muffin trays, and then bake for twenty-five minutes. Serve warm.

Nutrition:

- Calories: 316
- Protein: 11.2 g
- Fat: 14.5 g
- Carbs: 36.8 g
- Sodium: 469 mg
- Cholesterol: 43 mg

Berry Quinoa Bowls

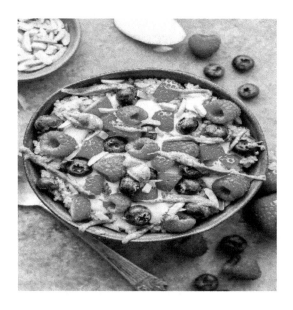

Preparation Time: 15 minutes

Cooking Time: 20 minutes

Servings: 2

Ingredients:

- 1 small peach, sliced
- 2/3 + ¾ cup milk, low fat
- 1/3 cup uncooked quinoa, rinsed well
- ½ teaspoon vanilla extract, pure
- 2 teaspoons brown sugar
- 14 blueberries
- 2 teaspoons honey, raw
- 12 raspberries

Directions:

1. Start to boil your quinoa, vanilla, 2/3 cup milk, and brown sugar together for five minutes before reducing it to a simmer. Cook for twenty minutes.
2. Heat a grill pan that's been greased over medium heat, and then add in your peaches to grill for one minute per side.
3. Heat the remaining ¾ cup of milk in your microwave. Cook the quinoa with a splash of milk, berries, and grilled peaches. Don't forget to drizzle with honey before serving it.

Nutrition:

- Calories: 435
- Protein: 9.2 g
- Fat: 13.7 g
- Carbs: 24.9 g
- Sodium: 141 mg
- Cholesterol: 78 mg

Pineapple Green Smoothie

Preparation Time: 5 minutes

Cooking Time: 0 minutes

Servings: 2

Ingredients:

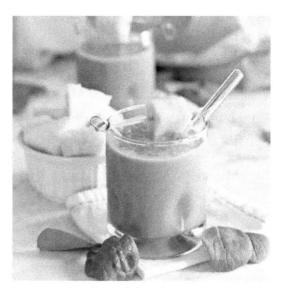

- 1 ¼ cups orange juice
- ½ cup Greek yogurt, plain
- 1 cup spinach, fresh
- 1 cup pineapple, frozen & chunked
- 1 cup mango, frozen & chunked
- 1 tablespoon ground flaxseed
- 1 teaspoon granulated stevia

Directions:

1. Start by blending everything together until smooth, and then serve cold.

Nutrition:

- Calories: 213
- Protein: 9 g
- Fat: 2 g
- Carbs: 43 g
- Sodium: 44 mg
- Cholesterol: 2.5 mg

Peanut Butter & Banana Smoothie

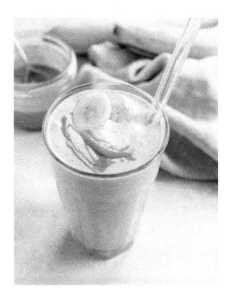

Preparation Time: 5 minutes

Cooking Time: 0 minutes

Servings: 1

Ingredients:

- 1 cup milk, nonfat
- 1 tablespoon peanut butter, all natural
- 1 banana, frozen & sliced

Directions:

1. Start by blending everything together until smooth.

Nutrition:

- Calories: 146
- Protein: 1.1 g
- Fat: 5.5 g
- Carbs: 1.8 g
- Sodium: 40 mg

Pumpkin-Hazelnut Tea Cake

Preparation Time: 5 minutes

Cooking Time: 55 minutes

Servings: 2

Ingredients:

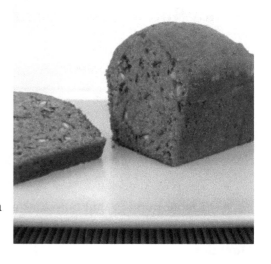

- 3 tablespoons canola oil
- 3/4 cup homemade or unsweetened canned pumpkin puree
- 1/2 cup honey
- 3 tablespoons firmly packed brown sugar
- 2 eggs, lightly beaten
- 1 cup whole-wheat (whole-meal) flour
- 1/2 cup all-purpose (plain) flour
- 2 tablespoons flaxseed
- 1/2 teaspoon baking powder
- 1/2 teaspoon ground allspice
- 1/2 teaspoon ground cinnamon
- 1/2 teaspoon ground nutmeg
- 1/4 teaspoon ground cloves
- 1/4 teaspoon salt
- 2 tablespoons chopped hazelnuts (filberts)

Directions:

1. Grease an 8x4 inch loaf pan with cooking spray. Set the oven to 350 degrees F.
2. Beat pumpkin puree with brown sugar, honey, eggs, and canola oil in a mixer.
3. Stir in flaxseed, allspice, baking powder, flours, cinnamon, cloves, salt, flours, and salt.
4. Mix well until it forms a smooth batter, transfer this batter to the loaf pan. Top it evenly with hazelnuts.
5. Press the nuts down, then bake for 55 minutes.
6. Allow the bread to cool for 10 minutes.
7. Slice and serve.

Nutrition:

- Calories 166
- Total Fat 6.5 g
- Cholesterol 43 mg
- Sodium 469 mg
- Total Carbs 27.8 g
- Protein 11.2 g

Raspberry Chocolate Scones

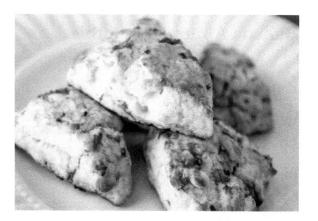

Preparation Time: 7 minutes

Cooking Time: 12 minutes

Servings: 2

Ingredients:

- 1 cup whole-wheat pastry flour
- 1 cup all-purpose flour
- 1 tablespoon baking powder
- 1/4 teaspoon baking soda
- 1/3 cup trans-fat-free buttery spread
- 1/2 cup fresh or frozen raspberries
- 1/4 cup miniature chocolate chips
- 1 cup plus 2 tablespoons plain fat-free yogurt
- 2 tablespoons honey
- 1/2 teaspoon sugar
- 1/4 teaspoon cinnamon

Directions:

1. Preheat the oven to 400 degrees F.
2. Combine flours with baking soda and baking powder in a mixing bowl.
3. Cut the butter into the dry mixture until it forms a crumbly mixture.
4. Fold in chocolate chips and berries.
5. Pour in honey and yogurt, then stir the mixture gently to form a crumbly batter.
6. Knead the dough ball on a surface, then spread it into ½ inch thick circle.
7. Slice the sheet into 12 wedges, then arrange them on a greased baking tray.
8. Sprinkle sugar and cinnamon mixture on top.
9. Bake them for 12 minutes at 400 degrees F.
10. Serve and enjoy.

Nutrition:

- Calories 149
- Total Fat 13.7 g
- Cholesterol 78 mg
- Sodium 141 mg
- Total Carbs 22.9 g
- Fiber 3.2 g
- Sugar 1.3 g
- Protein 4.2 g

Banana Almond Smoothie

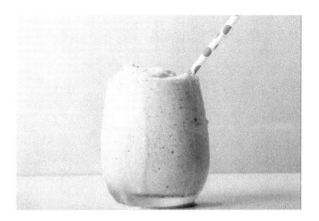

Preparation Time: 3 minutes

Cooking Time: 0 minutes

Servings: 2

Ingredients:

- 10 ounces (2 large) banana, frozen
- 4 tablespoons flaxseeds
- 2 tablespoons almond butter
- 1 cup almond milk
- ½ teaspoon honey
- ¼ teaspoon vanilla extract

Directions:

1. Using a blender, combine all the ingredients, until it becomes smooth.
2. Transfer the entire mix into two serving glass.
3. Serve fresh or refrigerate and consume.

Nutrition:

- Calories: 581
- Total Fat: 42.5 g
- Total Carbs: 47.5 g
- Dietary Fiber 11.7 g
- Cholesterol: 0 mg
- Sodium: 25 mg
- Protein: 10.3 g

Blueberry Banana Muffins

Preparation Time: 20 minutes

Cooking Time: 25 minutes

Serving: 2

Ingredients:

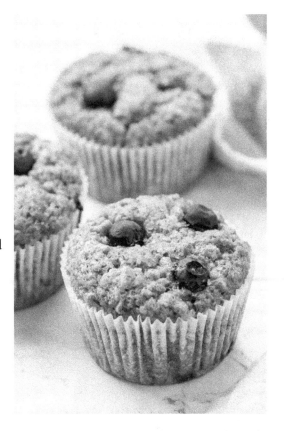

- 20 ounces (4 large) ripe banana, mashed
- 1¼ cups blueberries, fresh or frozen
- ¾ cup+2 tablespoons almond milk, unsweetened
- ¼ cup maple syrup
- 1 teaspoon apple cider vinegar
- 1 teaspoon vanilla extract
- 2 cups white flour
- ¼ cup coconut oil
- 2 teaspoons baking powder
- 6 tablespoons cane sugar
- 1½ teaspoons cinnamon, ground
- ½ teaspoon baking soda
- ½ teaspoon salt - ½ cup walnut halves, chopped

Directions:

1. Set the oven to 360°F and preheat. Spray some cooking oil into the muffin tin.
2. In a standard-sized bowl, mash all bananas and take ¾ cup. Refrigerate the remaining portion for making the smoothie. Put the mashed banana into a bowl along with the vinegar, milk, maple syrup, and vanilla. Do not stir. In a big bowl, mix all the dry ingredients like sugar, flour, cinnamon, baking powder, salt, and baking soda.
3. Stir in coconut oil into the dry mixture and combine well.
4. Pour all wet items mentioned in step 4 on top of the dry ingredients and blend them. Avoid over mixing. Put walnuts into the mix and after that the blueberries, and make sure that you have not over mix the ingredients. Over mixing may make it like a thick batter and the muffin become strong and spoil the dish. Spoon ¼ cup of batter into every tin of muffin, Bake the muffin at 370°F for 22 to 27 minutes. Insert a toothpick to check its baking status. When inserted the toothpick, it should come out clean. After baking is over, keep it 5-8 minutes to settle down and transfer to the cooling rack, keep it there for 15 minutes. Serve fresh.

Nutrition:

- Calories: 296 Total Carbohydrates: 36.3 g Dietary Fiber: 1.7 g Sugars: 16.4 g
- Total Fat: 14.6 g Cholesterol: 0 mg Sodium: 161 mg Protein: 3.9 g

Easy Buckwheat Crepes

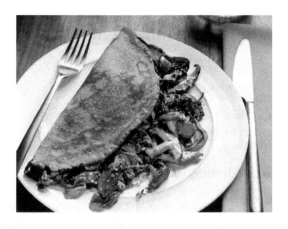

Preparation Time: 10 minutes

Cooking Time: 15 minutes

Serving: 2

Ingredients:

For making Crepes:

- 1 cup buckwheat flour, raw, un-toasted
- 1¾ cups light coconut milk, low-fat
- ¾ tablespoon flaxseed
- 1 tablespoon melted coconut oil
- ⅛ teaspoon ground cinnamon
- ⅛ teaspoon salt
- ⅛ teaspoon stevia

For fillings:

- 8 tablespoons nut butter
- 6 tablespoons granola
- 6 tablespoons compote
- 8 tablespoons -coconut whipped cream
- 3 cinnamon baked apples

Directions:

1. Put buckwheat flour, flaxseed, light coconut milk, coconut oil, salt, cinnamon, and stevia into a blender. Blend the above ingredients until it combines well. Blend until it turns into a pourable batter. Add a little buckwheat flour if the dough is too thin. If the batter is too thick, add some dairy-free milk.
2. Heat a nonstick skillet on medium temperature. Once, the skillet is hot, spread some oil in the bottom evenly. When the oiled surface of the skillet becomes hot, pour ¼ cup of batter into the skillet and cook until the top turns bubbly and the edges become dry. Carefully flip the crepes to cook for 2 minutes more. Do not let the skillet become too hot. Repeat the process until you finish all the crepes. To keep the warmness of the crepes, keep parchment paper between the crepes.
3. Serve it with vegan butter, or maple syrup or nut butter, or coconut whipped cream or cinnamon banked apples. You can also serve it with bananas or berries.
4. It's best if you serve it fresh, but you can easily store leftovers sealed in the refrigerator for up to 3 days. You can use it after reheating.

Nutrition:

- Calories: 230 Total Fat: 16.6 g Total Carbs: 24.6 g Dietary Fiber: 3.2 g
- Total Sugars: 3 g Cholesterol: 0 mg Sodium: 39 mg Protein: 4.2 g

Peanut Butter Oats in the Jar

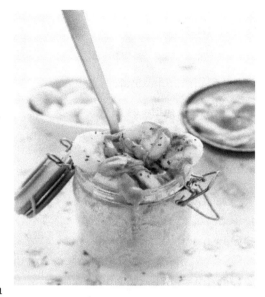

Preparation Time: 6 hours and 5 minutes

Cooking Time: 0 minutes

Servings: 1

Ingredients

For the oats:

- ½ cup gluten-free rolled oats
- ½ cup unsweetened, plain almond milk
- 4 tablespoons natural salted peanut butter
- 1 tablespoon maple syrup (or stevia, organic brown sugar)
- ¾ tablespoon chia seeds

For the toppings (optional):

- Banana, sliced
- Strawberries or raspberries
- Chia seeds

Directions:

1. Combine the almond milk, peanut butter, chia seeds, and maple syrup in a Mason jar. Stir but don't over-mix to leave swirls of peanut butter. Add the oats and stir again.
2. Press down the oats with a spoon to make sure they are soaked in the milk mixture.
3. Secure the jar with a lid and refrigerate for at least 6 hours.
4. To serve, garnish with toppings of choice.

Note: Nutritional info does not include toppings.

Nutrition:

- Calories: 454
- Carbohydrates: 50.9g
- Fat: 3.9g
- Fiber: 12g
- Protein: 14.6g
- Sodium: 162mg
- Sugar: 14.9g

Fruit Smoothie

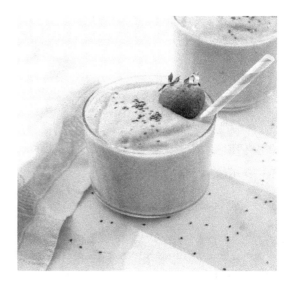

Preparation Time: 5 minutes

Cooking Time: 5 minutes

Servings: 1

Ingredients:

- One-fourth cup blueberries
- Four oz. strawberries
- One-half orange, peeled
- Four oz. papaya peeled, seeded, and diced
- One-fourth cup ice cubes
- Four oz. soy milk

Directions:

1. Pulse the blueberries, strawberries, peeled orange, and milk in a blender for approximately half a minute.
2. Combine the ice cubes and papaya and continue to blend for another 30 seconds.
3. Transfer to a glass and enjoy immediately.
4. You can also use frozen fruit if you prefer.

Nutrition:

- Sodium: 71 mg
- Protein: 6 g
- Fat: 3 g
- Sugar: 26 g
- Calories: 184
- Carbs: 43 g

Green Smoothie

Preparation Time: 5 minutes

Cooking Time: 5 minutes

Servings: 1

Ingredients:

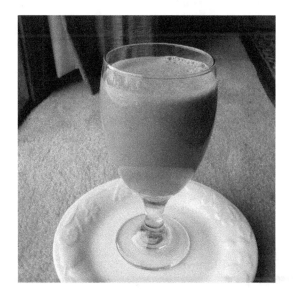

- One-fourth cup yogurt, non-fat and plain
- One-half tsp. vanilla extract
- One cup spinach
- One medium banana
- One-half cup milk, fat-free
- Three-fourths cup mango
- One-fourth cup whole oats

Directions:

1. Using a blender, combine the baby spinach, yogurt, whole oats, milk, and mango. Pulse for approximately half a minute.
2. Blend the banana and vanilla extract and pulse for an additional half minute until smooth.
3. Empty into a serving glass and enjoy immediately.

Nutrition:

- Sodium: 20 mg
- Protein: 2 g
- Fat: 0 g
- Sugar: 5 g
- Calories: 48
- Carbs: 38 g

Heart-Friendly Sweet Potato-Oats Waffles

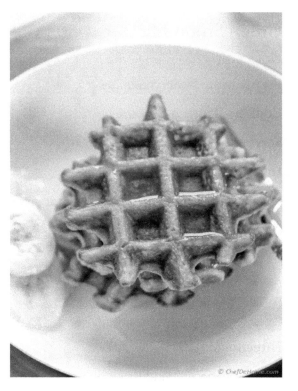

Preparation Time: 5 minutes

Cooking Time: 10 minutes

Servings: 2

Ingredients:

For the waffles:

- 1 cup rolled oats
- ½ cup Sweet potato, cooked and skin removed
- 1 whole egg
- 1 egg white
- 1 cup almond milk
- 1 tablespoon honey
- 1 tablespoon olive oil
- ¼ teaspoon baking powder
- ¼ teaspoon salt

To serve:

- Banana, sliced
- Maple syrup

Directions:

1. Preheat the waffle iron.
2. Meanwhile, add all the ingredients to a blender and process until pureed. Let the mixture rest for 10 minutes.
3. Coat the waffle iron with a nonstick cooking spray.
4. Pour ⅓ cup of the batter into each mold. Cook about 3-4 minutes per batch or 30 seconds longer after the light indicator turns green. Usually, waffles are done after the steam stops coming out of the waffle iron.
5. Serve with banana slices and maple syrup on top.

Nutrition:

- Calories: 287 Carbohydrates: 54g
- Fat: 8.39g Fiber: 7.2g
- Protein: 12.42g
- Sodium: 285mg
- Sugar: 22g

Rhubarb Pecan Muffins

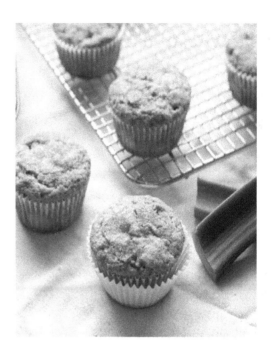

Preparation Time: 10 minutes

Cooking Time: 30 minutes

Servings: 2

Ingredients:

- 1 cup all-purpose (plain) flour
- 1 cup whole-wheat (whole-meal) flour
- 1/2 cup sugar
- 1 1/2 teaspoon baking powder
- 1/2 teaspoon baking soda
- 1/2 teaspoon salt
- 2 egg whites
- 2 tablespoons canola oil
- 2 tablespoons unsweetened applesauce
- 2 teaspoons grated orange peel
- 3/4 cup calcium-fortified orange juice
- 1 1/4 cup finely chopped rhubarb
- 2 tablespoons chopped pecans

Directions:

1. Set the oven to heat at 350 degrees F. Layer a muffin pan with muffin paper.
2. Combine flours with baking soda, baking powder, sugar, and salt in a bowl.
3. Whisk egg whites with orange peel, orange juice, applesauce, and canola oil in another container.
4. Add this wet mixture to the dry ingredients and mix well until smooth.
5. Fold in chopped rhubarb, then divide the mixture into the muffin cups.
6. Top the batter with a ½ teaspoon with chopped pecans.
7. Bake the muffin for 30 minutes then allow them to cool.
8. Serve.

Nutrition:

- Calories 143
- Total Fat 15.5 g
- Cholesterol 0 mg
- Sodium 31 mg
- Total Carbs 21.8 g
- Fiber 2.6 g
- Sugar 4.5 g
- Protein 4.1 g

Whole-Wheat Pretzels

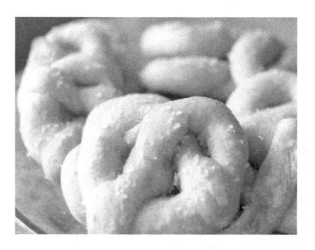

Preparation Time: 10 minutes

Cooking Time: 15 minutes

Servings: 2

Ingredients:

- 1 package active dry yeast
- 2 teaspoons brown sugar
- 1/2 teaspoon kosher salt
- 1 1/2 cups warm water
- 1 cup bread flour
- 3 cups whole-wheat flour
- 1 tablespoon olive oil
- 1/2 cup wheat gluten
- Cooking spray, as needed
- 1/4 cup baking soda
- 1 egg white or 1/4 cup egg substitute
- 1 tablespoon of sesame, poppy, or sunflower seeds

Directions:

1. Preheat the oven to 450 degrees F.
2. Mix yeast with salt, sugar, and water in a bowl and let it rest for 5 minutes.
3. Combine flours with gluten and olive oil in a processor.
4. Mix in the yeast mixture and knead the dough until smooth.
5. Cover the dough in the bowl with a plastic sheet and keep it in a warm place for 1 hour until the dough has raised.
6. Now, punch down the dough and divide the dough into 14 pieces.
7. Roll each piece into long ropes and make a pretzel shape out of this dough rope.
8. Boil 10 cups of water with ¼ cup baking soda in a pot. Place the pretzels in the water.
9. Cook each pretzel for 30 seconds then immediately transfer them to a baking pan lined with parchment paper using a slotted spoon.
10. Brush each pretzel with whisked egg whites and drizzle sesame, sunflower, and poppy seeds on top.
11. Bake them for 15 minutes at 450 degrees F
12. Serve.

Nutrition:

- Calories 148 Total Fat 12.8 g
- Cholesterol 112 mg Sodium 32 mg
- Total Carbs 31.5 g Fiber 4.2 g Sugar 2.5 g Protein 7.6 g

Mushroom Frittata

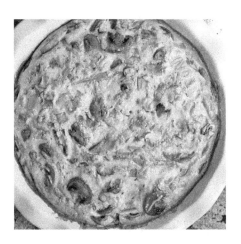

Preparation Time: 15 minutes

Cooking Time: 10 minutes

Servings: 2

Ingredients:

- 4 shallots, chopped
- 1 tablespoons butter
- 2 teaspoons parsley, fresh & diced
- ½ lb. mushrooms, fresh & diced
- 3 eggs
- 1 teaspoon thyme
- 5 egg whites
- ¼ teaspoon black pepper
- 1 tablespoon half & half, fat-free
- ¼ cup parmesan cheese, grated

Directions:

1. Start by turning the oven to 350, and then get out a skillet. Grease it with butter, letting it melt over medium heat.
2. Once your butter is hot adding in your shallots. Cook until golden brown, which should take roughly five minutes.
3. Stir in your thyme, pepper, parsley, and mushrooms.
4. Beat your eggs, egg whites, parmesan, and half and half together in a bowl.
5. Pour the mixture over your mushrooms, cooking for two minutes. Transfer the skillet to the oven, and bake for fifteen minutes. Slice to serve warm.

Nutrition:

- Calories: 391
- Protein: 7.6 g
- Fat: 12.8 g
- Carbs: 31.5 g
- Sodium: 32 mg
- Cholesterol: 112 mg

Cheesy Omelet

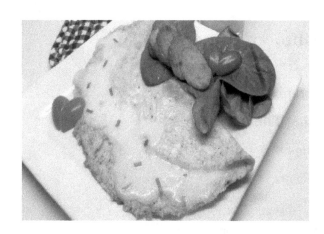

Preparation Time: 10 minutes

Cooking Time: 10 minutes

Servings: 2

Ingredients:

- 4 eggs
- 4 cups broccoli florets
- 1 tablespoon olive oil
- 1 cup egg whites
- ¼ cup cheddar, reduced-fat
- ¼ cup romano, grated
- ¼ teaspoon sea salt, fine
- ¼ teaspoon black pepper
- Cooking spray as needed

Directions:

1. Start by heating your oven to 350, and then steam your broccoli over boiling water for five to seven minutes. It should be tender.
2. Mash the broccoli into small pieces, and then toss with salt, pepper, and olive oil.
3. Get out a muffin tray and then grease it with cooking spray. Divide your broccoli between the cups, and then get out a bowl.
4. In the bowl beat your eggs with salt, pepper, egg whites, and parmesan.
5. Pour your batter over the broccoli, and then top with cheese. Bake for two minutes before serving warm.

Nutrition:

- Calories: 427
- Protein: 7.5 g
- Fat: 8.6 g
- Carbs: 13 g
- Sodium: 282 mg
- Cholesterol: 4.2 g

Ginger Congee

Preparation Time: 10 minutes

Cooking Time: 1 hour

Servings: 1

Ingredients:

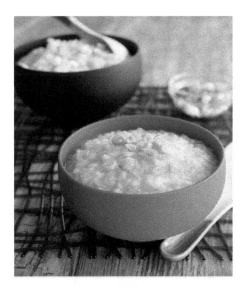

- 1 cup white rice, long grain & rinsed
- 7 cups chicken stock
- 1 inch ginger, peeled & sliced thin
- green onion, sliced for garnish
- sesame seed oil to garnish

Directions:

1. Start by boiling your ginger, rice, and salt in a pot. Allow it to simmer and reduce to low heat. Give it a gentle stir, and then allow it to cook for an hour. It should be thick and creamy.
2. Garnish by drizzling with sesame oil and serving warm.

Nutrition:

- Calories: 510
- Protein: 13.5 g
- Carbs: 60.7 g
- Fat: 24.7 g
- Sodium: 840 mg
- Cholesterol: 0 mg

Egg Melts

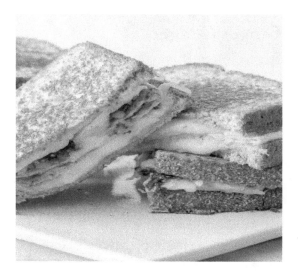

Preparation Time: 10 minutes

Cooking Time: 10 minutes

Servings: 2

Ingredients:

- 1 teaspoon olive oil
- 2 English muffins, whole grain & split
- 4 scallions, sliced fine
- 8 egg whites, whisked
- ¼ teaspoon sea salt, fine
- ¼ teaspoon black pepper
- ½ cup Swiss cheese, shredded & reduced fat
- ½ cup grape tomatoes, quartered

Directions:

1. Set the oven to broil, and then put your English muffins on a baking sheet. Make sure the split side is facing up. Broil for two minutes. They should turn golden around the edges.
2. Get out a skillet and grease with oil. Place it over medium heat, and cook your scallions for three minutes.
3. Beat your egg whites with salt and pepper, and pour this over your scallions.
4. Cook for another minute, stirring gently.
5. Spread this on your muffins, and top with remaining scallions if desired, cheese and tomatoes. Broil for 1 and a half more minutes to melt the cheese and serve warm.

Nutrition:

- Calories: 212
- Protein: 5.3 g
- Fat: 3.9 g
- Carbs: 14.3 g
- Sodium: 135 mg
- Cholesterol: 0 mg

CHAPTER 17:

Salads

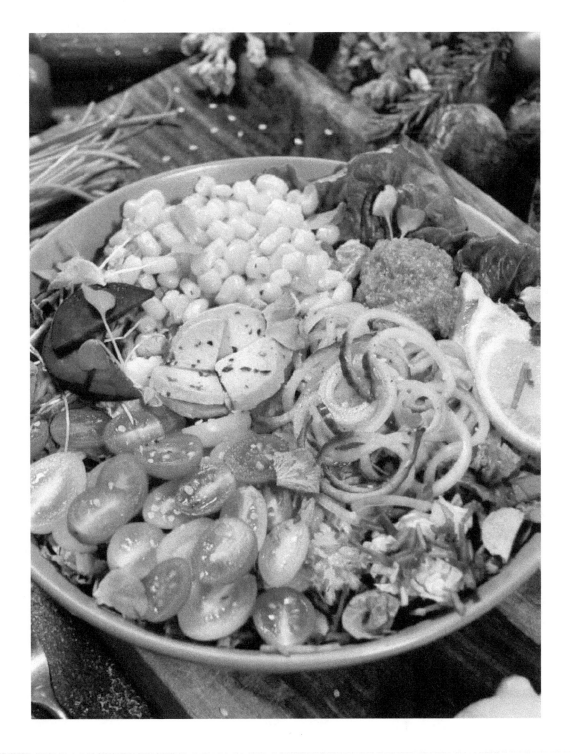

Spring Greens Salad

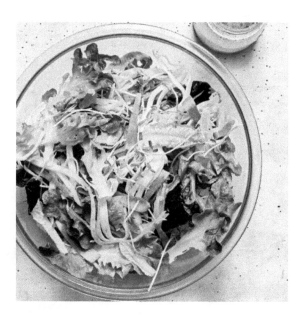

Preparation Time: 5 minutes

Cooking Time: 0 minutes

Servings: 2

Ingredients:

- ½ cup radish, sliced
- 1 cup fresh spinach, chopped
- ½ cup green peas, cooked
- ½ lemon
- 1 cup arugula, chopped
- 1 tablespoon avocado oil
- ½ teaspoon dried sage

Directions:

1. In the salad bowl, mix up radish, spinach, green peas, arugula, and dried sage.
2. Then squeeze the lemon over the salad.
3. Add avocado oil and shake the salad.

Nutrition:

- 54 calories
- 3.1g protein
- 9g carbohydrates
- 1.3g fat
- 3.6g fiber
- 0 mg cholesterol

Tuna Salad

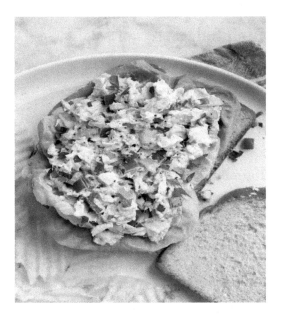

Preparation Time: 7 minutes

Cooking Time: 0 minutes

Servings: 2

Ingredients:

- ½ cup low-fat Greek yogurt
- 8 oz tuna, canned
- ½ cup fresh parsley, chopped
- 1 cup corn kernels, cooked
- ½ teaspoon ground black pepper

Directions:

1. Mix up tuna, parsley, kernels, and ground black pepper.
2. Then add yogurt and stir the salad until it is homogenous.

Nutrition:

- 172 calories
- 17.8g protein
- 13.6g carbohydrates
- 5.5g fat
- 1.4g fiber
- 19mg cholesterol
- 55mg sodium

Fish Salad

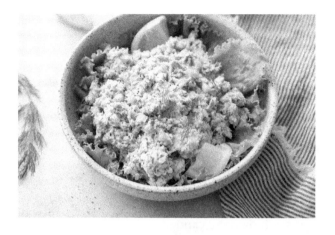

Preparation Time: 5 minutes

Cooking Time: 0 minutes

Servings: 2

Ingredients:

- 7 oz canned salmon, shredded
- 1 tablespoon lime juice
- 1 tablespoon low-fat yogurt
- 1 cup baby spinach, chopped
- 1 teaspoon capers, drained and chopped

Directions:

1. Mix up all ingredients together and transfer them into the salad bowl.

Nutrition:

- 71 calories
- 10.1g protein
- 0.8g carbohydrates
- 3.2g fat
- 0.2g fiber
- 22mg cholesterol
- 52mg sodium

Salmon Salad

Preparation Time: 10 minutes

Cooking Time: 0 minutes

Servings: 2

Ingredients:

- 4 oz canned salmon, flaked
- 1 tablespoon lemon juice
- 2 tablespoons red bell pepper, chopped
- 1 tablespoon red onion, chopped
- 1 teaspoon dill, chopped
- 1 tablespoon olive oil

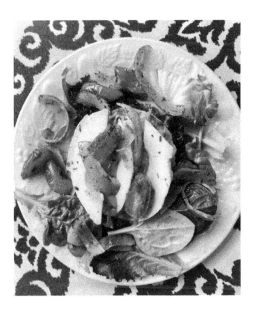

Directions:

1. Mix up all ingredients in the salad bowl.

Nutrition:

- 119 calories
- 8.3g protein
- 6.6g carbohydrates
- 7.3g fat
- 1.2g fiber
- 17mg cholesterol
- 21mg sodium

Arugula Salad with Shallot

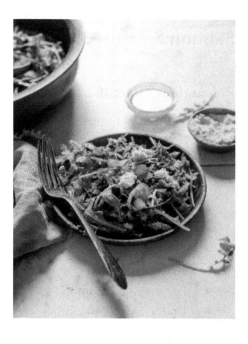

Preparation Time: 10 minutes

Cooking Time: 0 minutes

Servings: 2

Ingredients:

- 1 cup cucumber, chopped
- 1 tablespoon lemon juice
- 1 tablespoon avocado oil
- 2 shallots, chopped
- ½ cup black olives, sliced
- 3 cups arugula, chopped

Directions:

1. Mix up all ingredients from the list above in the salad bowl and refrigerate in the fridge for 5 minutes.

Nutrition:

- 33 calories
- 0.8g protein
- 2.9g carbohydrates
- 2.4g fat
- 1.1g fiber
- 0mg cholesterol
- 152mg sodium

Watercress Salad

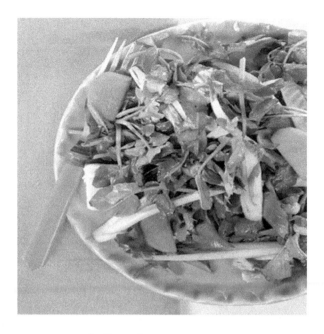

Preparation Time: 10 minutes

Cooking Time: 4 minutes

Servings: 2

Ingredients:

- 2 cups asparagus, chopped
- 16 ounces shrimp, cooked
- 4 cups watercress, torn
- 1 tablespoon apple cider vinegar
- ¼ cup olive oil

Directions:

1. In the mixing bowl mix up asparagus, shrimps, watercress, and olive oil.

Nutrition:

- 264 calories
- 28.3g protein
- 4.5g carbohydrates
- 14.8g fat
- 1.8g fiber
- 239mg cholesterol
- 300mg sodium

Seafood Arugula Salad

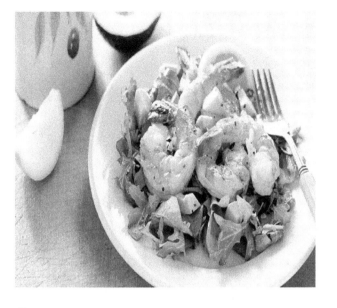

Preparation Time: 5 minutes

Cooking Time: 10 minutes

Servings: 2

Ingredients:

- 1 tablespoon olive oil
- 2 cups shrimps, cooked
- 1 cup arugula
- 1 tablespoon cilantro, chopped

Directions:

1. Put all ingredients in the salad bowl and shake well.

Nutrition:

- 61 calories
- 6.6g protein
- 0.2g carbohydrates
- 3.7g fat
- 0.1g fiber
- 123mg cholesterol
- 216mg sodium

Smoked Salad

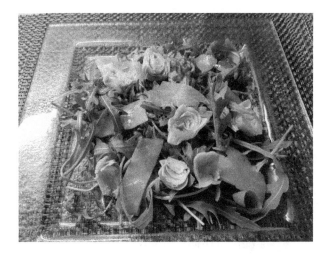

Preparation Time: 10 minutes

Cooking Time: 0 minutes

Servings: 2

Ingredients:

- 1 mango, chopped
- 4 cups lettuce, chopped
- 8 oz smoked turkey, chopped
- 2 tablespoons low-fat yogurt
- 1 teaspoon smoked paprika

Directions:

1. Mix up all ingredients in the bowls and transfer them to the serving plates.

Nutrition:

- 88 calories
- 7.1g protein
- 11.2g carbohydrates
- 1.9g fat
- 1.3g fiber
- 25mg cholesterol
- 350mg sodium

Avocado Salad

Preparation Time: 5 minutes

Cooking Time: 0 minutes

Servings: 2

Ingredients:

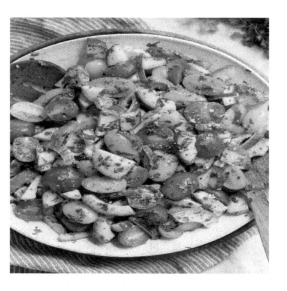

- ½ teaspoon ground black pepper
- 1 avocado, peeled, pitted and sliced
- 4 cups lettuce, chopped
- 1 cup black olives, pitted and halved
- 1 cup tomatoes, chopped
- 1 tablespoon olive oil

Directions:

1. Put all ingredients in the salad bowl and mix up well.

Nutrition:

- 197 calories
- 1.9g protein
- 10g carbohydrates
- 17.1g fat
- 5.4g fiber
- 0mg cholesterol
- 301mg sodium

Berry Salad with Shrimps

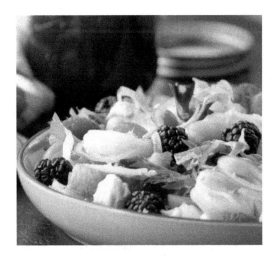

Preparation Time: 7 minutes

Cooking Time: 0 minutes

Servings: 2

Ingredients:

- 1 cup corn kernels, cooked
- 1 endive, shredded
- 1 pound shrimp, cooked
- 1 tablespoon lime juice
- 2 cups raspberries, halved
- 2 tablespoons olive oil
- 1 tablespoon parsley, chopped

Directions:

1. Put all ingredients from the list above in the salad bowl and shake well.

Nutrition:

- 283 calories
- 29.5g protein
- 21.2g carbohydrates
- 10.1g fat
- 9.1g fiber
- 239mg cholesterol
- 313mg sodium

Sliced Mushrooms Salad

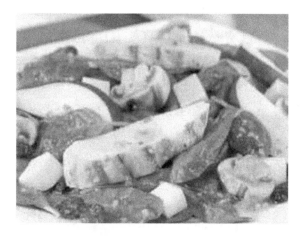

Preparation Time: 10 minutes

Cooking Time: 20 minutes

Servings: 2

Ingredients:

- 1 cup mushrooms, sliced
- 1 tablespoon margarine
- 1 cup lettuce, chopped
- 1 teaspoon lemon juice
- 1 tablespoon fresh dill, chopped
- 1 teaspoon cumin seeds

Directions:

2. Melt the margarine in the skillet.
3. Add mushrooms and lemon juice. Sauté the vegetables for 20 minutes over medium heat.
4. Then transfer the cooked mushrooms to the salad bowl, add lettuce, dill, and cumin seeds.
5. Stir the salad well.

Nutrition:

- 35 calories
- 0.9g protein
- 1.7g carbohydrates
- 3.1g fat
- 0.5g fiber
- 0mg cholesterol
- 38mg sodium

Tender Green Beans Salad

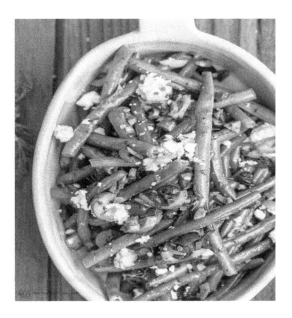

Preparation Time: 5 minutes

Cooking Time: 0 minutes

Servings: 2

Ingredients:

- 2 cups green beans, trimmed, chopped, cooked
- 2 tablespoons olive oil
- 2 pounds shrimp, cooked, peeled
- 1 cup tomato, chopped
- ¼ cup apple cider vinegar

Directions:

1. Mix up all ingredients together.
2. Then transfer the salad to the salad bowl.

Nutrition:

- 179 calories
- 26.5g protein
- 4.6g carbohydrates
- 5.5g fat
- 1.2g fiber
- 239mg cholesterol
- 280mg sodium

Spinach and Chicken Salad

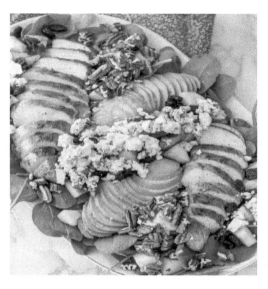

Preparation Time: 7 minutes

Cooking Time: 0 minutes

Servings: 2

Ingredients:

- 1 tablespoon olive oil
- A pinch of black pepper
- 1-pound chicken breast, cooked, skinless, boneless, shredded
- 1 pound cherry tomatoes, halved
- 1 red onion, sliced
- 3 cups spinach, chopped
- 1 tablespoon lemon juice
- 1 tablespoon nuts, chopped

Directions:

1. Put all ingredients in the salad bowl and gently stir with the help of a spatula.

Nutrition:

- 209 calories
- 26.4g protein
- 8.4g carbohydrates
- 7.8g fat
- 2.7g fiber
- 73mg cholesterol
- 97mg sodium

Cilantro Salad

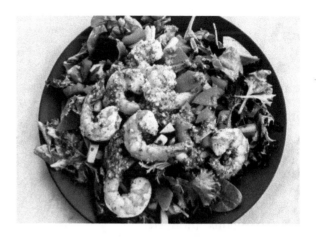

Preparation Time: 10 minutes

Cooking Time: 8 minutes

Servings: 2

Ingredients:

- 1 tablespoon avocado oil
- 1 pound shrimp, peeled and deveined
- 2 cups lettuce, chopped
- 1 tablespoon balsamic vinegar
- 1 tablespoon lemon juice
- 1 cup fresh cilantro, chopped

Directions:

1. Heat up a pan with the oil over medium heat, add the shrimps and cook them for 4 minutes per side or until they are light brown.
2. Transfer the shrimps to the salad bowl and add all remaining ingredients from the list above. Shake the salad.

Nutrition:

- 146 calories
- 26.1g protein
- 3g carbohydrates
- 2.5g fat
- 0.5g fiber
- 239mg cholesterol
- 281mg sodium

Iceberg Salad

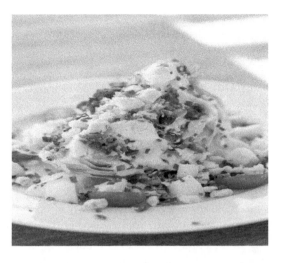

Preparation Time: 10 minutes

Cooking Time: 0 minutes

Servings: 2

Ingredients:

- 1 cup iceberg lettuce, chopped
- 2 oz scallions, chopped
- 1 cup carrot, shredded
- 1 cup radish, sliced
- 2 tablespoons red vinegar
- ¼ cup olive oil

Directions:

1. Make the dressing: mix up olive oil and red vinegar.
2. Then mix up all remaining ingredients in the salad bowl.
3. Sprinkle the salad with dressing.

Nutrition:

- 130 calories
- 0.8g protein
- 5.1g carbohydrates
- 12.7g fat
- 1.6g fiber
- 0mg cholesterol
- 33mg sodium

Seafood Salad with Grapes

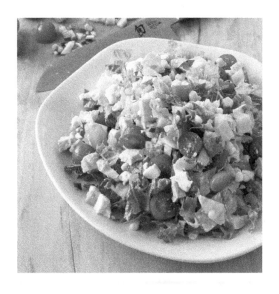

Preparation Time: 5 minutes

Cooking Time: 0 minutes

Servings: 2

Ingredients:

- 2 tablespoons low-fat mayonnaise
- 2 teaspoons chili powder
- 1-pound shrimp, cooked, peeled
- 1 cup green grapes, halved
- 1 oz nuts, chopped

Directions:

1. Mix up all ingredients in the mixing bowl and transfer the salad to the serving plates.

Nutrition:

- 225 calories
- 27.4g protein
- 9.9g carbohydrates
- 8.3g fat
- 1.3g fiber
- 241mg cholesterol
- 390mg sodium

CHAPTER 18:

Soups & Stews

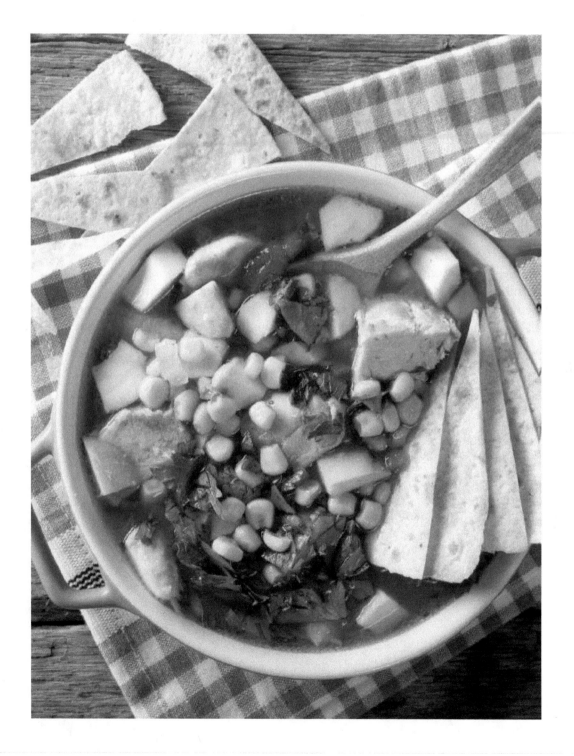

Pumpkin Cream Soup

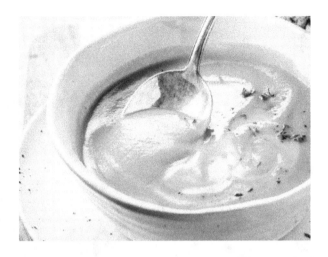

Preparation Time: 10 minutes

Cooking Time: 20 minutes

Servings: 2

Ingredients:

- 1-pound pumpkin, chopped
- 1 teaspoon ground cumin
- ½ cup cauliflower, chopped
- 4 cups of water
- 1 teaspoon ground turmeric
- ½ teaspoon ground nutmeg
- 1 tablespoon fresh dill, chopped
- 1 teaspoon olive oil
- ½ cup skim milk

Directions:

1. Roast the pumpkin with olive oil in the saucepan for 3 minutes.
2. Then stir well and add cauliflower, cumin, turmeric, nutmeg, and water.
3. Close the lid and cook the soup on medium mode for 15 minutes or until the pumpkin is soft.
4. Then blend the mixture until smooth and add skim milk. Remove the soup from heat and top with dill.

Nutrition:

- 56 calories
- 2.2g protein
- 10g carbohydrates
- 1.4g fat
- 3.1g fiber
- 0mg cholesterol
- 28mg sodium

Zucchini Noodles Soup

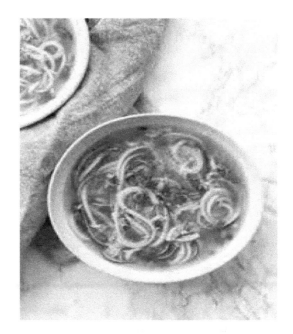

Preparation Time: 10 minutes

Cooking Time: 15 minutes

Servings: 2

Ingredients:

- 2 zucchinis, trimmed
- 4 cups low-sodium chicken stock
- 2 oz fresh parsley, chopped
- ½ teaspoon chili flakes
- 1 oz carrot, shredded
- 1 teaspoon canola oil

Directions:

1. Roast the carrot with canola oil in the saucepan for 5 minutes over medium-low heat.
2. Stir it well and add chicken stock. Bring the mixture to a boil.
3. Meanwhile, make the noodles from the zucchini with the help of the spiralizer.
4. Add them to the boiling soup liquid.
5. Add parsley and chili flakes. Bring the soup to a boil and remove it from the heat.
6. Leave for 10 minutes to rest.

Nutrition:

- 39 calories
- 2.7g protein
- 4.9g carbohydrates
- 1.5g fat
- 1.7g fiber
- 0mg cholesterol
- 158mg sodium

Grilled Tomatoes Soup

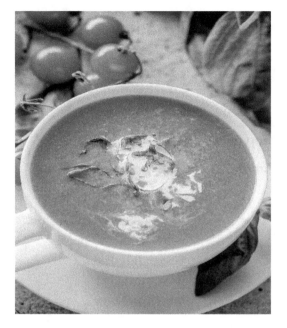

Preparation Time: 10 minutes

Cooking Time: 20 minutes

Servings: 1

Ingredients:

- 2-pounds tomatoes
- ½ cup shallot, chopped
- 1 tablespoon avocado oil
- ½ teaspoon ground black pepper
- ¼ teaspoon minced garlic
- 1 tablespoon dried basil
- 3 cups low-sodium chicken broth

Directions:

1. Cut the tomatoes into halves and grill them in the preheated to 390F grill for 1 minute from each side.
2. After this, transfer the grilled tomatoes to the blender and blend until smooth.
3. Place the shallot and avocado oil in the saucepan and roast it until light brown.
4. Add blended grilled tomatoes, ground black pepper, and minced garlic.
5. Bring the soup to a boil and sprinkle with dried basil.
6. Simmer the soup for 2 minutes more.

Nutrition:

- 72 calories
- 4.1g protein
- 13.4g carbohydrates
- 0.9g fat
- 3g fiber
- 0mg cholesterol
- 98mg sodium

Chicken Oatmeal Soup

Preparation Time: 10 minutes

Cooking Time: 15 minutes

Servings: 2

Ingredients:

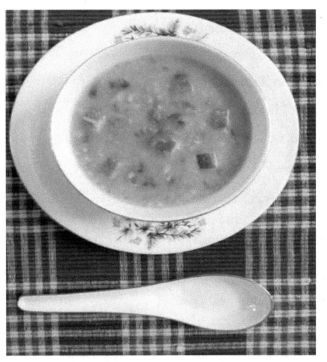

- 1 cup oats
- 4 cups of water
- 1 oz fresh dill, chopped
- 10 oz chicken fillet, chopped
- 1 teaspoon ground black pepper
- 1 teaspoon potato starch
- ½ carrot, diced

Directions:

1. Put the chopped chicken in the saucepan, add water, and bring it to a boil. Simmer the chicken for 10 minutes.
2. Add dill, ground black pepper, oats, and diced carrot.
3. Bring the soup to a boil and add potato starch. Stir it until the soup starts to thicken. Simmer the soup for 5 minutes on low heat.

Nutrition:

- 192 calories
- 19.8g protein
- 16.1g carbohydrates
- 5.5g fat
- 2.7g fiber
- 50mg cholesterol
- 72mg sodium

Celery Cream Soup

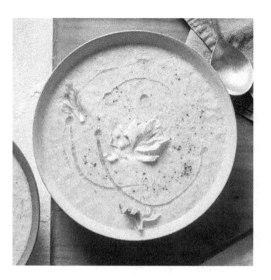

Preparation Time: 10 minutes

Cooking Time: 25 minutes

Servings: 1

Ingredients:

- 2 cups celery stalk, chopped
- 1 shallot, chopped
- 1 potato, chopped
- 4 cups low-sodium vegetable stock
- 1 tablespoon margarine
- 1 teaspoon white pepper

Directions:

1. Melt the margarine in the saucepan, add shallot, and celery stalk. Cook the vegetables for 5 minutes. Stir them occasionally.
2. After this, add vegetable stock and potato.
3. Simmer the soup for 15 minutes.
4. Blend the soup until you get the creamy texture and sprinkle with white pepper.
5. Simmer it for 5 minutes more.

Nutrition:

- 88 calories
- 2.3g protein
- 13.3g carbohydrates
- 3g fat
- 2.9g fiber
- 0mg cholesterol
- 217mg sodium
- 449mg potassium

Cauliflower Soup

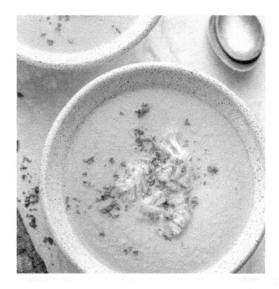

Preparation Time: 10 minutes

Cooking Time: 20 minutes

Servings: 2

Ingredients:

- 1 cup cauliflower, chopped
- ¼ cup potato, chopped
- 1 cup skim milk
- 1 cup of water
- 1 teaspoon ground coriander
- 1 teaspoon margarine

Directions:

1. Put cauliflower and potato in the saucepan.
2. Add water and boil the ingredients for 15 minutes.
3. Then add ground coriander and margarine.
4. With the help of the immersion blender, blend the soup until smooth.
5. Add skim milk and stir well.

Nutrition:

- 82 calories
- 5.2g protein
- 10.3g carbohydrates
- 2g fat
- 1.5g fiber
- 2mg cholesterol
- 106mg sodium

Buckwheat Soup

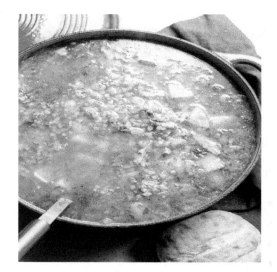

Preparation Time: 10 minutes

Cooking Time: 25 minutes

Servings: 2

Ingredients:

- ½ cup buckwheat
- 1 carrot, chopped
- 1 yellow onion, diced
- 1 tablespoon avocado oil
- 1 tablespoon fresh dill, chopped
- 1-pound chicken breast, chopped
- 1 teaspoon ground black pepper
- 6 cups of water

Directions:

1. Sauté the onion, carrot, and avocado oil in the saucepan for 5 minutes. Stir them from time to time.
2. Then add buckwheat, chicken breast, and ground black pepper.
3. Add water and close the lid.
4. Simmer the soup for 20 minutes.
5. After this, add dill and remove the soup from the heat. Leave it for 10 minutes to rest.

Nutrition:

- 152 calories
- 18.4g protein
- 13.5g carbohydrates
- 2.7g fat
- 2.3g fiber
- 48mg cholesterol
- 48mg sodium

Parsley Soup

Preparation Time: 10 minutes

Cooking Time: 16 minutes

Servings: 2

Ingredients:

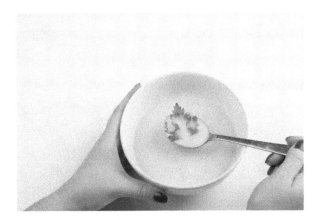

- 2 teaspoons olive oil
- 1 cup carrot, shredded
- 1 cup yellow onion, chopped
- 1 cup celery, chopped
- 6 cups of water
- 1 cup fresh parsley, chopped
- ¼ cup low-fat parmesan, grated

Directions:

1. Heat up a pot with the oil over medium-high heat, add onion, carrot, and celery, stir and cook for 7 minutes.
2. Add water and all remaining ingredients.
3. Cook the soup for 8 minutes over medium heat.

Nutrition:

- 46 calories
- 1.6g protein
- 4.8g carbohydrates
- 2.5g fat
- 1.5g fiber
- 4mg cholesterol
- 103mg sodium

Tomato Bean Soup

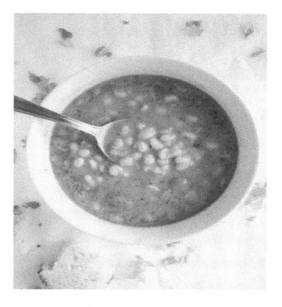

Preparation Time: 10 minutes

Cooking Time: 25 minutes

Servings: 1

Ingredients:

- 2 teaspoons olive oil
- 2 garlic cloves, minced
- 1 pound green beans, trimmed and halved
- 4 tomatoes, cubed
- 1 teaspoon sweet paprika
- 4 cup of water
- 2 tablespoons dill, chopped

Directions:

1. Heat up a pot with the oil over medium-high heat, add the garlic stir. Sauté the garlic for 5 minutes.
2. Add all remaining ingredients and cook the soup for 20 minutes.

Nutrition:

- 57 calories
- 2.4g protein
- 9.7g carbohydrates
- 1.9g fat
- 3.8g fiber
- 0mg cholesterol
- 16mg sodium

Red Kidney Beans Soup

Preparation Time: 10 minutes

Cooking Time: 20 minutes

Servings: 2

Ingredients:

- 2 teaspoons olive oil
- 1 yellow onion, chopped
- 1 teaspoon cinnamon powder
- 1 cup red kidney beans, cooked
- 3 cups low-sodium chicken broth
- 1 potato, chopped

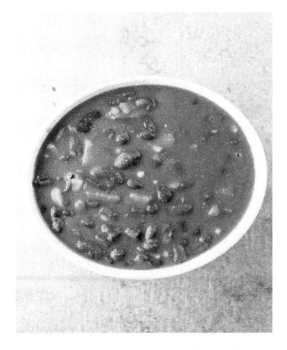

Directions:

1. Heat up a pot with the oil over medium heat, add onion and cinnamon, stir and cook for 6 minutes.
2. Add all remaining ingredients and cook them for 14 minutes.
3. Blend the soup until you get a puree texture.

Nutrition:

- 230 calories
- 13g protein
- 38.9g carbohydrates
- 2.9g fat
- 8.5g fiber
- 0mg cholesterol
- 62mg sodium

Pork Soup

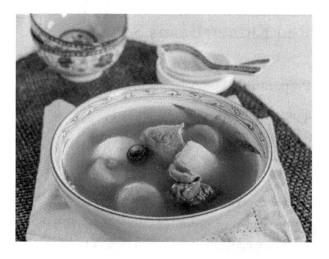

Preparation Time: 10 minutes

Cooking Time: 25 minutes

Servings: 2

Ingredients:

- 1 tablespoon avocado oil
- 1 onion, chopped
- 1 pound pork stew meat, cubed
- 4 cups of water
- 1 pound carrots, sliced
- 1 teaspoon tomato paste

Directions:

1. Heat up a pot with the oil over medium-high heat, add the onion and pork, and cook the ingredients for 5 minutes.
2. Add all remaining ingredients and cook the soup for 20 minutes.

Nutrition:

- 304 calories
- 34.5g protein
- 14.2g carbohydrates
- 11.4g fat
- 3.6g fiber
- 98mg cholesterol
- 155mg sodium

Curry Soup

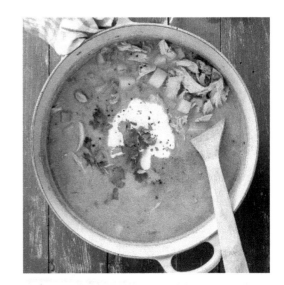

Preparation Time: 10 minutes

Cooking Time: 23 minutes

Servings: 2

Ingredients:

- 3 tablespoons olive oil
- 8 carrots, peeled and sliced
- 2 teaspoons curry paste
- 4 celery stalks, chopped
- 1 yellow onion, chopped
- 4 cups of water

Directions:

1. Heat up a pot with the oil and add onion, celery and carrots, stir and cook for 12 minutes.
2. Then add curry paste and water. Stir the soup well and cook it for 10 minutes more.
3. When all ingredients are soft, blend the soup until smooth and simmer it for 1 minute more.

Nutrition:

- 171 calories
- 1.6g protein
- 15.8g carbohydrates
- 12g fat
- 3.9g fiber
- 0mg cholesterol
- 106mg sodium

Yellow Onion Soup

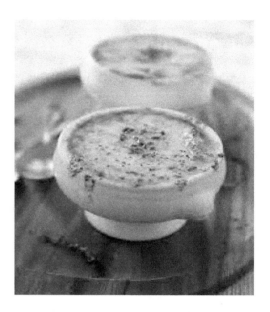

Preparation Time: 10 minutes

Cooking Time: 20 minutes

Servings: 2

Ingredients:

- 1 tablespoon avocado oil
- 1 yellow onion, chopped
- 1 teaspoon ginger, grated
- 1 pound zucchinis, chopped
- 4 cups low-sodium chicken broth
- ½ cup low-fat cream
- 1 teaspoon ground black pepper

Directions:

1. Heat up a pot with the oil over medium heat, add the onion and ginger, stir and cook for 5 minutes.
2. Add all remaining ingredients and simmer them over medium heat for 15 minutes.
3. Blend the cooked soup and ladle in the bowls.

Nutrition:

- 61 calories
- 4.2g protein
- 10.2g carbohydrates
- 0.7g fat
- 2.2g fiber
- 1mg cholesterol
- 101mg sodium

Garlic Soup

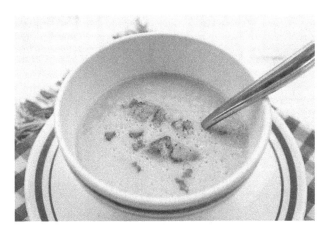

Preparation Time: 10 minutes

Cooking Time: 50 minutes

Servings: 2

Ingredients:

- 1 pound red kidney beans, cooked
- 8 cups of water
- 1 green bell pepper, chopped
- 1 tomato paste
- 1 yellow onion, chopped
- 1 teaspoon minced garlic
- 1 pound beef sirloin, cubed
- 1 teaspoon garlic powder

Directions:

1. Pour water into a pot and heat up over medium heat.
2. Add all ingredients and close the lid.
3. Simmer the soup for 45 minutes over medium heat.

Nutrition:

- 620 calories
- 60.9g protein
- 75.8g carbohydrates
- 8.4g fat
- 18.5g fiber
- 101mg cholesterol
- 109mg sodium

CHAPTER 19:

Vegan & Vegetarian

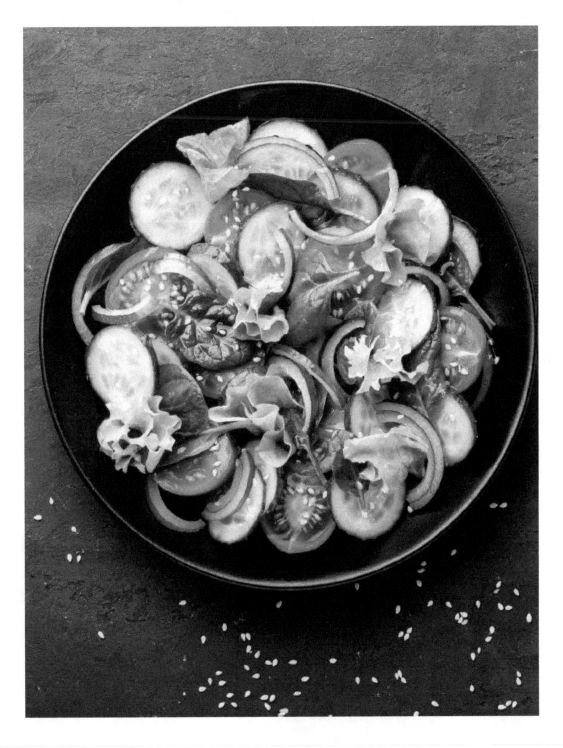

Chickpea Curry

Preparation Time: 10 minutes

Cooking Time: 10 minutes

Servings: 2

Ingredients:

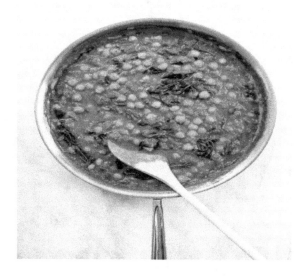

- 1 ½ cup chickpeas, boiled
- 1 teaspoon curry powder
- ½ teaspoon garam masala
- 1 cup spinach, chopped
- 1 teaspoon coconut oil
- ¼ cup of soy milk
- 1 tablespoon tomato paste
- ½ cup of water

Directions:

1. Heat up coconut oil in the saucepan.
2. Add curry powder, garam masala, tomato paste, and soy milk.
3. Whisk the mixture until smooth and bring it to a boil.
4. Add water, spinach, and chickpeas.
5. Stir the meal and close the lid.
6. Cook it for 5 minutes over medium heat.

Nutrition:

- 298 calories
- 15.4g protein
- 47.8g carbohydrates
- 6.1g fat
- 13.6g fiber
- 0mg cholesterol
- 37mg sodium

Quinoa Bowl

Preparation Time: 15 minutes

Cooking Time: 15 minutes

Servings: 1

Ingredients:

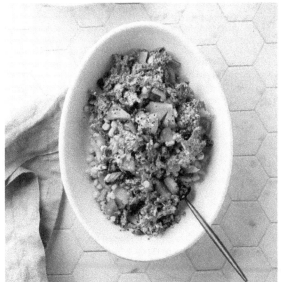

- 1 cup quinoa
- 2 cups of water
- 1 cup tomatoes, diced
- 1 cup sweet pepper, diced
- ½ cup of rice, cooked
- 1 tablespoon lemon juice
- ½ teaspoon lemon zest, grated
- 1 tablespoon olive oil

Directions:

1. Mix up water and quinoa and cook it for 15 minutes. Then remove it from the heat and leave to rest for 10 minutes.
2. Transfer the cooked quinoa to the big bowl.
3. Add tomatoes, sweet pepper, rice, lemon juice, lemon zest, and olive oil.
4. Stir the mixture well and transfer to the serving bowls.

Nutrition:

- 290 calories
- 8.4g protein
- 49.9g carbohydrates
- 6.4g fat
- 4.3g fiber
- 0mg cholesterol
- 11mg sodium

Vegan Meatloaf

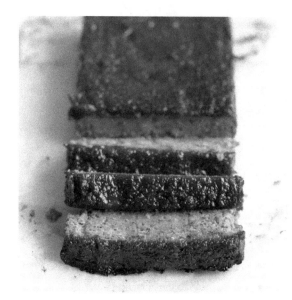

Preparation Time: 10 minutes

Cooking Time: 30 minutes

Servings: 2

Ingredients:

- 1 cup chickpeas, cooked
- 1 onion, diced
- 1 tablespoon ground flax seeds
- ½ teaspoon chili flakes
- 1 tablespoon coconut oil
- ½ cup carrot, diced
- ½ cup celery stalk, chopped
- 1 tablespoon tomato paste

Directions:

1. Heat up coconut oil in the saucepan.
2. Add carrot, onion, and celery stalk. Cook the vegetables for 8 minutes or until they are soft.
3. Then add chickpeas, chili flakes, and ground flax seeds.
4. Blend the mixture until smooth with the help of the immersion blender.
5. Then line the loaf mold with baking paper and transfer the blended mixture inside.
6. Flatten it well and spread with tomato paste.
7. Bake the meatloaf in the preheated to 365F oven for 20 minutes.

Nutrition:

- 162 calories
- 7.1g protein
- 23.9g carbohydrates
- 4.7g fat
- 7g fiber
- 0mg cholesterol
- 25mg sodium

Loaded Potato Skins

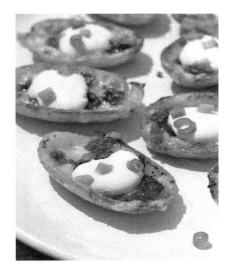

Preparation Time: 15 minutes

Cooking Time: 45 minutes

Servings: 2

Ingredients:

- 6 potatoes
- 1 teaspoon ground black pepper
- 2 tablespoons olive oil
- ½ teaspoon minced garlic
- ¼ cup of soy milk

Directions:

1. Preheat the oven to 400F.
2. Pierce the potatoes with the help of the knife 2-3 times and bake in the oven for 30 minutes or until the vegetables are tender.
3. After this, cut the baked potatoes into halves and scoop out the potato meat in the bowl.
4. Sprinkle the scooped potato halves with olive oil and ground black pepper and return them back to the oven. Bake them for 15 minutes or until they are light brown.
5. Meanwhile, mash the scooped potato meat and mix it up with soy milk and minced garlic.
6. Fill the cooked potato halves with the mashed potato mixture.

Nutrition:

- 194 calories
- 4g protein
- 34.4g carbohydrates
- 5.1g fat
- 5.3g fiber
- 0mg cholesterol
- 18mg sodium

Vegan Shepherd Pie

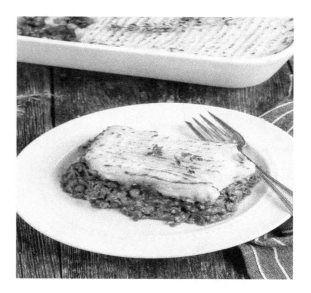

Preparation Time: 15 minutes

Cooking Time: 35 minutes

Servings: 2

Ingredients:

- ½ cup quinoa, cooked
- ½ cup tomato puree
- ½ cup carrot, diced
- 1 shallot, chopped
- 1 tablespoon coconut oil
- ½ cup potato, cooked, mashed
- 1 teaspoon chili powder
- ½ cup mushrooms, sliced

Directions:

1. Put carrot, shallot, and mushrooms in the saucepan.
2. Add coconut oil and cook the vegetables for 10 minutes or until they are tender but not soft.
3. Then mix up cooked vegetables with chili powder and tomato puree.
4. Transfer the mixture to the casserole mold and flatten well.
5. After this, top the vegetables with mashed potatoes. Cover the shepherd pie with foil and bake in the preheated to 375F oven for 25 minutes.

Nutrition:

- 136 calories
- 4.2g protein
- 20.1g carbohydrates
- 4.9g fat
- 2.9g fiber
- 0mg cholesterol
- 27mg sodium

Cauliflower Steaks

Preparation Time: 15 minutes

Cooking Time: 25 minutes

Servings: 2

Ingredients:

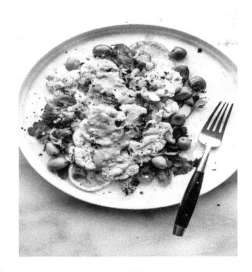

- 1-pound cauliflower head
- 1 teaspoon ground turmeric
- ½ teaspoon cayenne pepper
- 2 tablespoons olive oil
- ½ teaspoon garlic powder

Directions:

1. Slice the cauliflower head into the steaks and rub with ground turmeric, cayenne pepper, and garlic powder.
2. Then line the baking tray with baking paper and put the cauliflower steaks inside.
3. Sprinkle them with olive oil and bake at 375F for 25 minutes or until the vegetable steaks are tender.

Nutrition:

- 92 calories
- 2.4g protein
- 6.8g carbohydrates
- 7.2g fat
- 3.1g fiber
- 0mg cholesterol
- 34mg sodium

Quinoa Burger

Preparation Time: 15 minutes

Cooking Time: 20 minutes

Servings: 2

Ingredients:

- 1/3 cup chickpeas, cooked
- ½ cup quinoa, cooked
- 1 teaspoon Italian seasonings
- 1 teaspoon olive oil
- ½ onion, minced

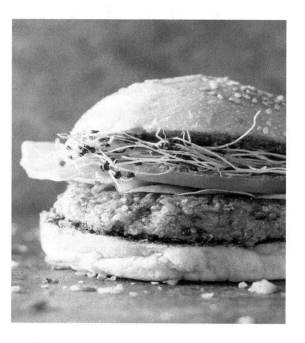

Directions:

1. Blend the chickpeas until they are smooth.
2. Then mix them up with quinoa, Italian seasonings, and minced onion. Stir the ingredients until homogenous.
3. After this, make the burgers from the mixture and place them in the lined baking tray.
4. Sprinkle the quinoa burgers with olive oil and bake them at 275F for 20 minutes.

Nutrition:

- 158 calories
- 6.4g protein
- 25.2g carbohydrates
- 3.8g fat
- 4.7g fiber
- 1mg cholesterol
- 6mg sodium

Cauliflower Tots

Preparation Time: 15 minutes

Cooking Time: 20 minutes

Servings: 1

Ingredients:

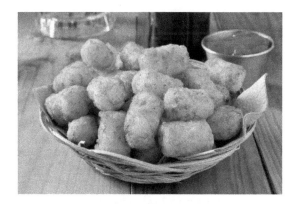

- 1 cup cauliflower, shredded
- 3 oz vegan Parmesan, grated
- 1/3 cup flax seeds meal
- 1 egg, beaten
- 1 teaspoon Italian seasonings
- 1 teaspoon olive oil

Directions:

1. In the bowl mix up shredded cauliflower, vegan Parmesan, flax seeds meal, egg, and Italian seasonings.
2. Knead the cauliflower mixture. Add water if needed.
3. After this, make the cauliflower tots from the mixture.
4. Line the baking tray with baking paper and place the cauliflower tots inside.
5. Sprinkle them with the olive oil and transfer in the preheated to 375F oven.
6. Bake the meal for 15-20 minutes or until golden brown.

Nutrition:

- 109 calories
- 6.1g protein
- 6.3g carbohydrates
- 6.6g fat
- 3.7g fiber
- 42mg cholesterol
- 72mg sodium

Zucchini Soufflé

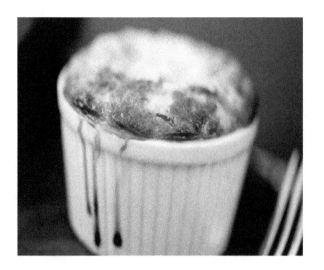

Preparation Time: 10 minutes

Cooking Time: 60 minutes

Servings: 2

Ingredients:

- 2 cups zucchini, grated
- ½ teaspoon baking powder
- ½ cup oatmeal, grinded
- 1 onion, diced
- 3 tablespoons water
- 1 teaspoon cayenne pepper
- 1 teaspoon dried thyme

Directions:

1. Mix up all ingredients together in the casserole mold.
2. Flatten well the zucchini mixture and cover with foil.
3. Bake the soufflé at 365F for 60 minutes.

Nutrition:

- 41 calories
- 1.6g protein
- 8.1g carbohydrates
- 0.6g fat
- 1.6g fiber
- 0mg cholesterol
- 6mg sodium

Honey Sweet Potato Bake

Preparation Time: 20 minutes

Cooking Time: 20 minutes

Servings: 2

Ingredients:

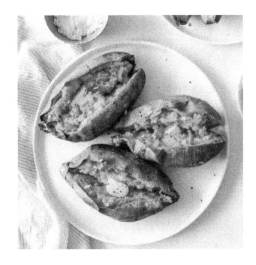

- 4 sweet potatoes, baked
- 1 tablespoon honey
- 1 teaspoon ground cinnamon
- ¼ teaspoon ground cardamom
- 1/3 cup soy milk

Directions:

1. Peel the sweet potatoes and mash them.
2. Then mix mashed potato with ground cinnamon, cardamom, and soy milk. Stir it well.
3. Transfer the mixture to the baking pan and flatten well.
4. Sprinkle the mixture with honey and cover with foil.
5. Bake the meal at 375F for 20 minutes.

Nutrition:

- 30 calories
- 0.7g protein
- 6.5g carbohydrates
- 0.4g fat
- 0.5g fiber
- 0mg cholesterol
- 11mg sodium

Lentil Quiche

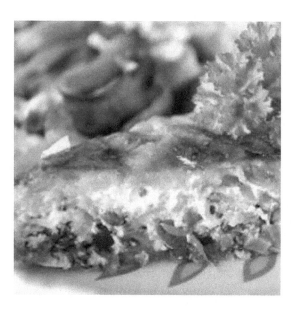

Preparation Time: 15 minutes

Cooking Time: 35 minutes

Servings: 2

Ingredients:

- 1 cup green lentils, boiled
- ½ cup carrot, grated
- 1 onion, diced
- 1 tablespoon olive oil
- ¼ cup flax seeds meal
- 1 teaspoon ground black pepper
- ¼ cup of soy milk

Directions:

1. Cook the onion with olive oil in the skillet until light brown.
2. Then mix up cooked onion, lentils, and carrot.
3. Add flax seeds meal, ground black pepper, and soy milk. Stir the mixture until homogenous.
4. After this, transfer it to the baking pan and flatten it.
5. Bake the quiche for 35 minutes at 375F.

Nutrition:

- 351 calories
- 17.1g protein
- 41.6g carbohydrates
- 13.1g fat
- 23.3g fiber
- 0mg cholesterol
- 29mg sodium

Corn Patties

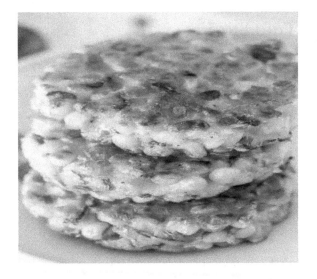

Preparation Time: 15 minutes

Cooking Time: 10 minutes

Servings: 1

Ingredients:

- ½ cup chickpeas, cooked
- 1 cup corn kernels, cooked
- 1 tablespoon fresh parsley, chopped
- 1 teaspoon chili powder
- ½ teaspoon ground coriander
- 1 tablespoon tomato paste
- 1 tablespoon almond meal
- 1 tablespoon olive oil

Directions:

1. Mash the cooked chickpeas and combine them with corn kernels, parsley, chili powder, ground coriander, tomato paste, and almond meal.
2. Stir the mixture until homogenous.
3. Make the small patties.
4. After this, heat up olive oil in the skillet.
5. Put the prepared patties in the hot oil and cook them for 3 minutes per side or until they are golden brown.
6. Dry the cooked patties with the help of paper towel if needed.

Nutrition:

- 168 calories
- 6.7g protein
- 23.9g carbohydrates
- 6.3g fat,
- 6g fiber
- 0mg cholesterol
- 23mg sodium

Tofu Stir Fry

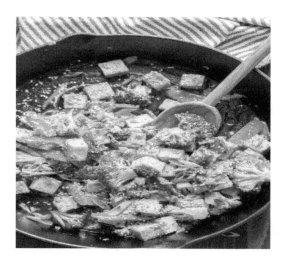

Preparation Time: 15 minutes

Cooking Time: 10 minutes

Servings: 2

Ingredients:

- 9 oz firm tofu, cubed
- 3 tablespoons low-sodium soy sauce
- 1 teaspoon sesame seeds
- 1 tablespoon sesame oil
- 1 cup spinach, chopped
- ¼ cup of water

Directions:

1. In the mixing bowl mix up soy sauce, and sesame oil.
2. Dip the tofu cubes in the soy sauce mixture and leave for 10 minutes to marinate.
3. Heat up a skillet and put the tofu cubes inside. Roast them for 1.5 minutes from each side.
4. Then add water, the remaining soy sauce mixture, and chopped spinach.
5. Close the lid and cook the meal for 5 minutes more.

Nutrition:

- 118 calories
- 8.5g protein
- 3.1g carbohydrates
- 8.6g fat
- 1.1g fiber
- 0mg cholesterol
- 406mg sodium

Mac Stuffed Sweet Potatoes

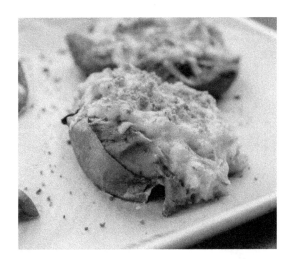

Preparation Time: 20 minutes

Cooking Time: 25 minutes

Servings: 2

Ingredients:

- 1 sweet potato
- ¼ cup whole-grain penne pasta
- 1 teaspoon tomato paste
- 1 teaspoon olive oil
- ¼ teaspoon minced garlic
- 1 tablespoon soy milk

Directions:

1. Cut the sweet potato in half and pierce it 3-4 times with the help of the fork.
2. Sprinkle the sweet potato halves with olive oil and bake in the preheated to 375F oven for 25-30 minutes or until the vegetables are tender.
3. Meanwhile, mix up penne pasta, tomato paste, minced garlic, and soy milk.
4. When the sweet potatoes are cooked, scoop out the vegetable meat and mix it up with a penne pasta mixture.
5. Fill the sweet potatoes with the pasta mixture.

Nutrition:

- 105 calories
- 2.7g protein
- 17.8g carbohydrates
- 2.8g fat
- 3g fiber
- 0mg cholesterol
- 28mg sodium

Tofu Tikka Masala

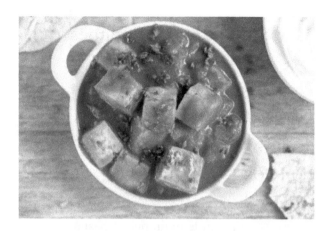

Preparation Time: 10 minutes

Cooking Time: 25 minutes

Servings: 2

Ingredients:

- 8 oz tofu, chopped
- ½ cup of soy milk
- 1 teaspoon garam masala
- 1 teaspoon olive oil
- 1 teaspoon ground paprika
- ½ cup tomatoes, chopped
- ½ onion, diced

Directions:

1. Heat up olive oil in the saucepan.
2. Add diced onion and cook it until light brown.
3. Then add tomatoes, ground paprika, and garam masala. Bring the mixture to a boil.
4. Add soy milk and stir well. Simmer it for 5 minutes.
5. Then add chopped tofu and cook the meal for 3 minutes.
6. Leave the cooked meal for 10 minutes to rest.

Nutrition:

- 155 calories
- 12.2g protein
- 20.7g carbohydrates
- 8.4g fat
- 2.9g fiber
- 0mg cholesterol
- 51mg sodium

Tofu Parmigiana

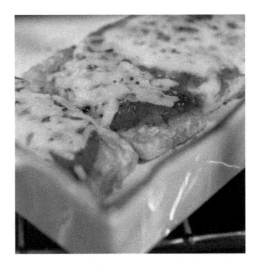

Preparation Time: 15 minutes

Cooking Time: 8 minutes

Servings: 2

Ingredients:

- 6 oz firm tofu, roughly sliced
- 1 teaspoon coconut oil
- 1 teaspoon tomato sauce
- ½ teaspoon Italian seasonings

Directions:

1. In the mixing bowl, mix up, tomato sauce, and Italian seasonings.
2. Then brush the sliced tofu with the tomato mixture well and leave for 10 minutes to marinate.
3. Heat up coconut oil.
4. Then put the sliced tofu in the hot oil and roast it for 3 minutes per side or until tofu is golden brown.

Nutrition:

- 83 calories
- 7g protein
- 1.7g carbohydrates
- 6.2g fat
- 0.8 fiber
- 1mg cholesterol
- 24mg sodium

Mushroom Stroganoff

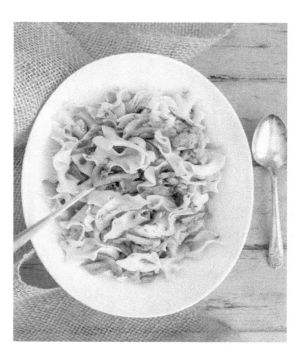

Preparation Time: 10 minutes

Cooking Time: 20 minutes

Servings: 2

Ingredients:

- 2 cups mushrooms, sliced
- 1 teaspoon whole-grain wheat flour
- 1 tablespoon coconut oil
- 1 onion, chopped
- 1 teaspoon dried thyme
- 1 garlic clove, diced
- 1 teaspoon ground black pepper
- ½ cup of soy milk

Directions:

- Heat up coconut oil in the saucepan.
- Add mushrooms and onion and cook them for 10 minutes. Stir the vegetables from time to time.
- After this, sprinkle them with ground black pepper, thyme, and garlic.
- Add soy milk and bring the mixture to a boil.
- Then add flour and stir it well until homogenous.
- Cook the mushroom stroganoff until it thickens.

Nutrition:

- 70 calories
- 2.6g protein
- 6.9g carbohydrates
- 4.1g fat
- 1.5g fiber
- 0mg cholesterol
- 19mg sodium

Eggplant Croquettes

Preparation Time: 15 minutes

Cooking Time: 5 minutes

Servings: 2

Ingredients:

- 1 eggplant, peeled, boiled
- 2 potatoes, mashed
- 2 tablespoons almond meal
- 1 teaspoon chili pepper
- 1 tablespoon coconut oil
- 1 tablespoon olive oil
- ¼ teaspoon ground nutmeg

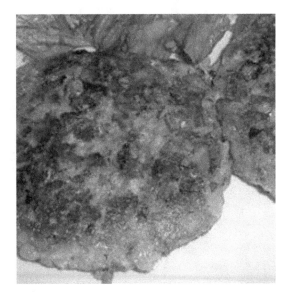

Directions:

1. Blend the eggplant until smooth.
2. Then mix it up with mashed potato, chili pepper, coconut oil, and ground nutmeg.
3. Make the croquettes from the eggplant mixture.
4. Heat up olive oil in the skillet.
5. Put the croquettes in the hot oil and cook them for 2 minutes per side or until they are light brown.

Nutrition:

- 180 calories
- 3.6g protein
- 24.3g carbohydrates
- 8.8g fat
- 7.1g fiber
- 0mg cholesterol
- 9mg sodium

Stuffed Portobello

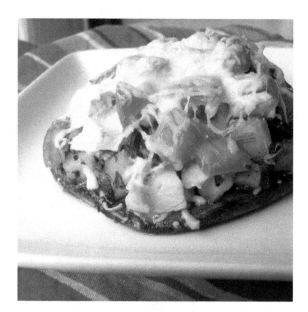

Preparation Time: 10 minutes

Cooking Time: 20 minutes

Servings: 2

Ingredients:

- 4 Portobello mushroom caps
- ½ zucchini, grated
- 1 tomato, diced
- 1 teaspoon olive oil
- ½ teaspoon dried parsley
- ¼ teaspoon minced garlic

Directions:

1. In the mixing bowl, mix up diced tomato, grated zucchini, dried parsley, and minced garlic.
2. Then fill the mushroom caps with zucchini mixture and transfer to the lined baking paper tray.
3. Bake the vegetables for 20 minutes or until they are soft.

Nutrition:

- 24 calories
- 1.2g protein
- 2.9g carbohydrates
- 1.3g fat
- 0.9g fiber
- 0mg cholesterol
- 5mg sodium

Chile Rellenos

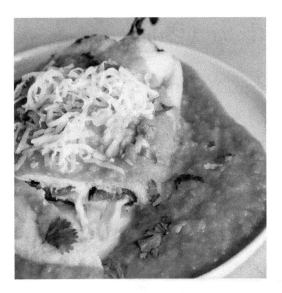

Preparation Time: 10 minutes

Cooking Time: 30 minutes

Servings: 2

Ingredients:

- 2 chili peppers
- 2 oz vegan Mozzarella cheese, shredded
- 2 oz tomato puree
- 1 tablespoon coconut oil
- 2 tablespoons whole-grain wheat flour
- 1 tablespoon potato starch
- ¼ cup of water
- ½ teaspoon chili flakes

Directions:

1. Bake the chili peppers for 15 minutes in the preheated to 375F oven.
2. Meanwhile, pour tomato puree into the saucepan.
3. Add chili flakes and bring the mixture to boil. Remove it from the heat.
4. After this, mix up potato starch, flour, and water.
5. When the chili peppers are cooked, make the cuts in them and remove the seeds.
6. Then fill the peppers with shredded cheese and secure the cuts with toothpicks.
7. Heat up coconut oil in the skillet.
8. Dip the chili peppers in the flour mixture and roast in the coconut oil until they are golden brown.
9. Sprinkle the cooked chilies with the tomato puree mixture.

Nutrition:

- 187 calories
- 4.2g protein
- 16g carbohydrates
- 12g fat
- 3.7g fiber
- 0mg cholesterol
- 122mg sodium

Garbanzo Stir Fry

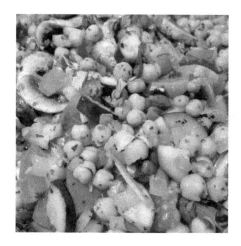

Preparation Time: 10 minutes

Cooking Time: 30 minutes

Ingredients:

Servings: 2

- 1 cup garbanzo beans, cooked
- 1 zucchini, diced
- 5 oz cremini mushrooms, chopped
- 1 tablespoon coconut oil
- 1 teaspoon ground black pepper
- 1 tablespoon fresh parsley, chopped
- 1 tablespoon lemon juice

Directions:

1. Heat up coconut oil in the saucepan.
2. Add mushrooms and roast them for 10 minutes.
3. Then add zucchini and cooked garbanzo beans. Stir the ingredients well and cook them for 10 minutes more.
4. After this, sprinkle the vegetables with ground black pepper and lemon juice. Cook the meal for 5 minutes.
5. Add parsley and mix it up. Cook it for 5 minutes more.

Nutrition:

- 231 calories
- 11.3g protein
- 33.9g carbohydrates
- 6.6g fat
- 9.6g fiber
- 0mg cholesterol
- 21mg sodium

CHAPTER 20:

Fish & Seafood

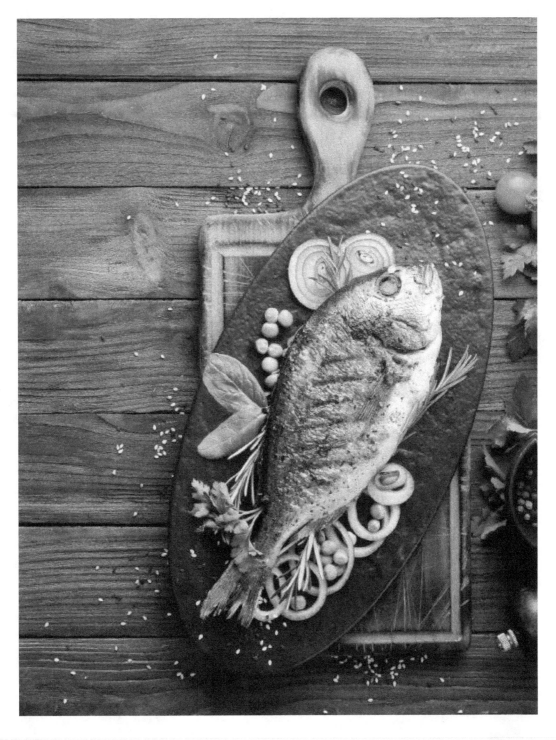

Halibut with Tomato, Basil, and Oregano Salsa

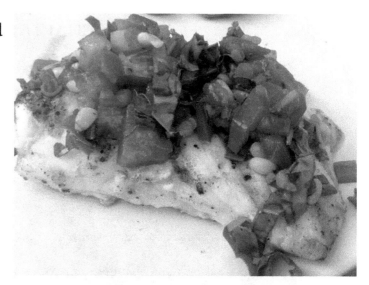

Preparation Time: 20 minutes

Cooking Time: 15 minutes

Servings: 2

Ingredients:

- Tomatoes - 2 diced
- Fresh basil - 2 tablespoons chopped
- Fresh oregano - 1 teaspoon chopped
- Garlic - 1 tablespoon minced
- Extra virgin olive oil - 2 teaspoons
- Halibut filets -4 ounces each
- Parmesan cheese - optional

Directions:

1. Preheat the oven to 350 °F (150 °C).
2. Lightly coat a glass 9 x 13-inch baking dish with cooking spray.
3. In a mixer, combine the tomato, basil, oregano, and garlic on chopping speed. Add the olive oil and chop for another minute to blend.
4. Arrange the halibut fillets in the baking dish. Pour the tomato mixture over the fish evenly. Place in the oven and bake for about 10 to 15 minutes.
5. Transfer to individual plates and spoon some of the tomato sauce over each fillet then serve immediately.
6. Sprinkle a little parmesan cheese over the top for an added kick of flavor.

Nutrition:

- Total fat 5 g
- Calories 160
- Protein 24 g
- Cholesterol 36 mg
- Total carbohydrate 3 g
- Dietary fiber 1 g
- Sodium 65 mg

Roasted Salmon with Chives and Tarragon

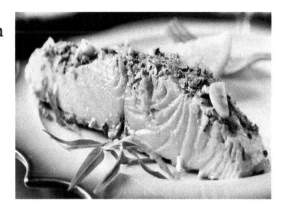

Preparation Time: 20 minutes

Cooking Time: 12 minutes

Servings: 2

Ingredients:

- Organic salmon with skin - 2 - 5 ounce pieces
- Extra virgin olive oil - 2 teaspoons
- Chives - 1 tablespoon chopped
- Fresh tarragon leaves - 1 teaspoon
- Cooking spray

Directions:

1. Preheat oven to 475 °F (250 °C).
2. Line a baking sheet with foil and light cooking spray.
3. Rub salmon with 2 teaspoons of extra virgin olive oil.
4. Roast skin side down about 12 minutes or until fish is thoroughly cooked.
5. Use a metal spatula to lift the salmon off the skin. Place salmon on the serving plate. Discard skin. Sprinkle salmon with herbs and serve.

Nutrition:

- Sodium 62 mg
- Total fat 14 g
- Cholesterol 78 mg
- Protein 28 g
- Calories 241
- Total carbohydrate 3.2 g

Grilled Shrimp Salad with Orange Vinaigrette

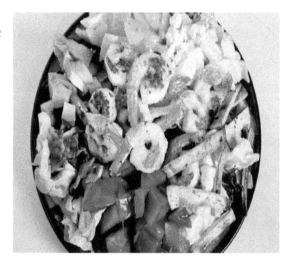

Preparation Time: 10 minutes

Cooking Time: 6 minutes

Servings: 2

Ingredients:

- 1 orange, juiced
- 1 lime, juiced
- 1 tsp fresh mint, chopped
- 1/2-lb. tail-on shrimps
- 1 small red onion, quartered
- 2 cups packed spinach leaves
- 1 avocado, peeled, seeded, and sliced
- 1 cup cherry tomatoes, sliced in half
- 1 orange, cut into segments

Directions:

1. In a small bowl, whisk well orange juice, lime juice, and mint.
2. In a medium bowl add shrimp a tbsp of the orange vinaigrette. Toss well to coat.
3. Skewer shrimps and red onion. Grill on preheated 400oF oven or grill for 4 minutes per side. Remove from grill and set aside to cool.
4. Evenly divide between two bowls the spinach leaves, avocado, cherry tomatoes, red onion, grilled shrimp, grilled onions, and orange segments.
5. Drizzle with vinaigrette, toss well to coat.
6. Serve and enjoy.

Nutrition:

- Calories: 351
- Protein: 27.7g
- Carbs: 31.0g
- Fat: 15.8g
- Saturated Fat: 2.3g
- Sodium: 172mg

Halibut with Radish Slices

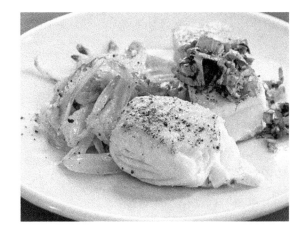

Preparation Time: 10 minutes

Cooking Time: 6 minutes

Servings: 2

Ingredients:

- 4 halibut fillets, boneless
- 1 cup radishes, sliced
- 1 tablespoon apple cider vinegar
- ¼ teaspoon ground coriander
- 1 tablespoon olive oil
- 1 teaspoon low-fat cream cheese

Directions:

1. Sprinkle the fish fillets with apple cider vinegar, ground coriander, and olive oil.
2. Then grill the halibut in the preheated to 385F grill for 3 minutes per side.
3. Transfer the fish to the plates and top with sliced radish and cream cheese.

Nutrition:

- 356 calories
- 60.8g protein
- 1g carbohydrates
- 10.5g fat
- 0.5g fiber
- 94mg cholesterol
- 170mg sodium

Green Onion Salmon

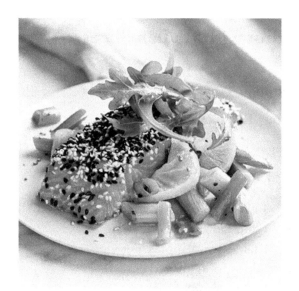

Preparation Time: 10 minutes

Cooking Time: 10 minutes

Servings: 2

Ingredients:

4 green olives, pitted, sliced

2 oz green onions, blended

½ teaspoon chili flakes

¼ teaspoon ground black pepper

3 tablespoons avocado oil

4 salmon fillets, skinless and boneless

1 oz parsley, chopped

Directions:

1. Blend together green onions, chili flakes, ground black pepper, avocado oil, and parsley.
2. Then rub the salmon fillets with green onion mixture and transfer them to the preheated skillet.
3. Cook it for 4 minutes per side.
4. Top the cooked fish with sliced olives.

Nutrition:

- 272 calories
- 35.1g protein
- 3.2g carbohydrates
- 13.4g fat
- 1.1g fiber
- 78mg cholesterol
- 375mg sodium

Broccoli and Cod Mash

Preparation Time: 10 minutes

Cooking Time: 20 minutes

Servings: 1

Ingredients:

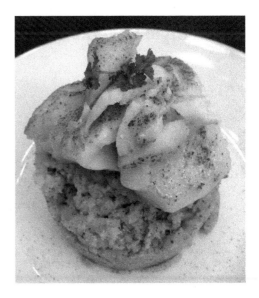

- 2 cups broccoli, chopped
- 4 cod fillets, boneless, chopped
- 1 white onion, chopped
- 2 tablespoons olive oil
- 1 cup of water
- 1 tablespoon low-fat cream cheese
- ½ teaspoon ground black pepper

Directions:

1. Roast the cod in the saucepan with olive oil for 1 minute per side.
2. Then add all remaining ingredients except cream cheese and boil the meal for 18 minutes.
3. After this, drain water, add cream cheese, and stir the meal well.

Nutrition:

- 186 calories
- 21.8g protein
- 5.8g carbohydrates
- 9.1g fat
- 1.8g fiber
- 43mg cholesterol
- 105mg sodium

Greek Style Salmon

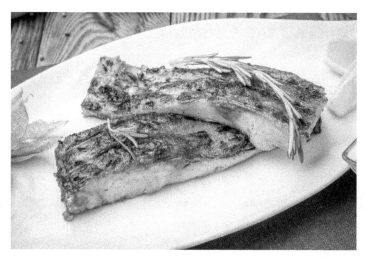

Preparation Time: 10 minutes

Cooking Time: 10 minutes

Servings: 2

Ingredients:

- 4 medium salmon fillets, skinless and boneless
- 1 tablespoon lemon juice
- 1 tablespoon dried oregano
- 1 teaspoon dried thyme
- ¼ teaspoon onion powder
- 1 tablespoon olive oil

Directions:

1. Heat up olive oil in the skillet.
2. Sprinkle the salmon with dried oregano, thyme, onion powder, and lemon juice.
3. Put the fish in the skillet and cook for 4 minutes per side.

Nutrition:

- 271 calories
- 34.7g protein
- 1.1g carbohydrates
- 14.7g fat
- 0.6g fiber
- 78mg cholesterol
- 80mg sodium

Spicy Ginger Seabass

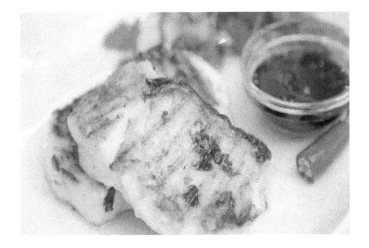

Preparation Time: 5 minutes

Cooking Time: 10 minutes

Servings: 2

Ingredients:

- 1 tablespoon ginger, grated
- 2 tablespoons sesame oil
- ¼ teaspoon chili powder
- 4 sea bass fillets, boneless
- 1 tablespoon margarine

Directions:

1. Heat up sesame oil and margarine in the skillet.
2. Add chili powder and ginger.
3. Then add seabass and cook the fish for 3 minutes per side.
4. Then close the lid and simmer the fish for 3 minutes over low heat.

Nutrition:

- 216 calories
- 24g protein
- 1.1g carbohydrates
- 12.3g fat
- 0.2g fiber
- 54mg cholesterol
- 123mg sodium

Yogurt Shrimps

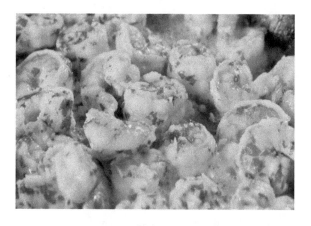

Preparation Time: 5 minutes

Cooking Time: 10 minutes

Servings: 2

Ingredients:

- 1 pound shrimp, peeled
- 1 tablespoon margarine
- ¼ cup low-fat yogurt
- 1 teaspoon lemon zest, grated
- 1 chili pepper, chopped

Directions:

1. Melt the margarine in the skillet, add chili pepper, and roast it for 1 minute.
2. Then add shrimps and lemon zest.
3. Roast the shrimps for 2 minutes per side.
4. After this, add yogurt, stir the shrimps well and cook for 5 minutes.

Nutrition:

- 137 calories
- 21.4g protein
- 2.4g carbohydrates
- 4g fat
- 0.1g fiber
- 192mg cholesterol
- 257mg sodium

Aromatic Salmon with Fennel Seeds

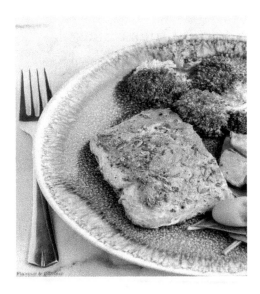

Preparation Time: 8 minutes

Cooking Time: 10 minutes

Servings: 2

Ingredients:

- 4 medium salmon fillets, skinless and boneless
- 1 tablespoon fennel seeds
- 2 tablespoons olive oil
- 1 tablespoon lemon juice
- 1 tablespoon water

Directions:

1. Heat up olive oil in the skillet.
2. Add fennel seeds and roast them for 1 minute.
3. Add salmon fillets and sprinkle with lemon juice.
4. Add water and roast the fish for 4 minutes per side over medium heat.

Nutrition:

- 301 calories
- 4.8g protein
- 0.8g carbohydrates
- 18.2g fat
- 0.6g fiber
- 78mg cholesterol
- 81mg sodium

Shrimp Quesadillas

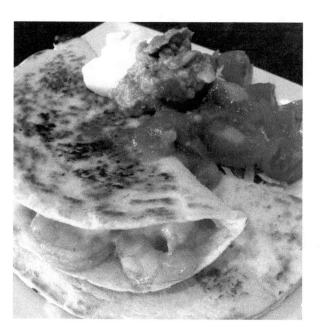

Preparation Time: 16 minutes

Cooking Time: 5 minutes

Servings: 2

Ingredients:

- Two whole wheat tortillas
- ½ tsp. ground cumin
- 4 cilantro leaves
- 3 oz. diced cooked shrimp
- 1 de-seeded plump tomato
- ¾ c. grated non-fat mozzarella cheese
- ¼ c. diced red onion

Directions:

1. In a medium bowl, combine the grated mozzarella cheese and the warm, cooked shrimp. Add the ground cumin, red onion, and tomato. Mix. Spread the mixture evenly on the tortillas.
2. Heat a non-stick frying pan. Place the tortillas in the pan, then heat until they crisp.
3. Add the cilantro leaves. Fold over the tortillas.
4. Press down for 1 – 2 minutes. Slice the tortillas into wedges.
5. Serve immediately.

Nutrition:

- Calories: 99
- Fat: 9 g
- Carbs: 7.2 g
- Protein: 59 g
- Sugars: 4 g
- Sodium: 500 mg

The OG Tuna Sandwich

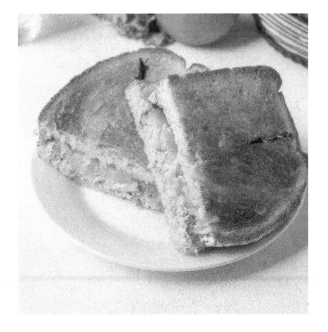

Preparation Time: 15 minutes

Cooking Time: 5 minutes

Servings: 2

Ingredients:

- 30 g olive oil
- 1 peeled and diced medium cucumber
- 2 ½ g pepper
- 4 whole-wheat bread slices
- 85 g diced onion
- 2 ½ g salt
- 1 can flavored tuna
- 85 g shredded spinach

Directions:

1. Grab your blender and add the spinach, tuna, onion, oil, salt, and pepper, and pulse for about 10 to 20 seconds.
2. In the meantime, toast your bread and add your diced cucumber to a bowl, which you can pour your tuna mixture in. Carefully mix and add the mixture to the bread once toasted.
3. Slice in half and serve, while storing the remaining mixture in the fridge.

Nutrition:

- Calories: 302
- Fat: 5.8 g
- Carbs: 36.62 g
- Protein: 28 g
- Sugars: 3.22 g
- Sodium: 445 mg

Easy To Make Mussels

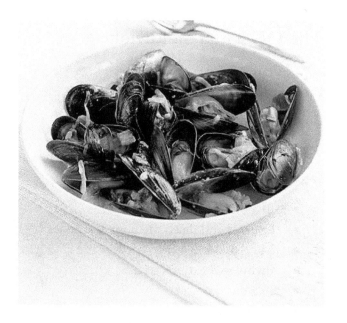

Preparation Time: 10 minutes

Cooking Time: 10 minutes

Servings: 2

Ingredients:

- 2 lbs. cleaned mussels
- 4 minced garlic cloves
- 2 chopped shallots
- Lemon and parsley
- 2 tbsps. Butter
- ½ c. broth
- ½ c. white wine

Directions:

1. Clean the mussels and remove the beard.
2. Discard any mussels that do not close when tapped against a hard surface.
3. Set your pot to Sauté mode and add chopped onion and butter.
4. Stir and sauté onions.
5. Add garlic and cook for 1 minute.
6. Add broth and wine.
7. Lock up the lid and cook for 5 minutes on HIGH pressure.
8. Release the pressure naturally over 10 minutes.
9. Serve with a sprinkle of parsley and enjoy!

Nutrition:

- Calories: 286
- Fat: 14 g
- Carbs: 12 g
- Protein: 28 g
- Sugars: 0 g
- Sodium: 314 mg

Chili-Rubbed Tilapia with Asparagus & Lemon

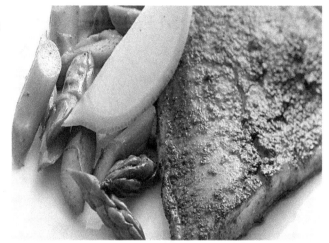

Preparation Time: 10 minutes

Cooking Time: 10 minutes

Servings: 2

Ingredients:

- 3 tbsps. lemon juice
- 2 tbsps. chili powder
- 2 tbsps. extra-virgin olive oil
- ½ tsp. divided salt
- 2 lbs. trimmed asparagus
- ½ tsp. garlic powder
- 1 lb. tilapia fillets

Directions:

1. Bring 1 inch of water to a boil in a large saucepan. Put asparagus in a steamer basket, place in the pan, cover, and steam until tender-crisp, about 4 minutes.
2. Transfer to a large plate, spreading out to cool.
3. Combine chili powder, garlic powder, and ¼ teaspoon salt on a plate. Dredge fillets in the spice mixture to coat. Heat oil in a large nonstick skillet over medium-high heat. Add the fish and cook until just opaque in the center, gently turning halfway, and 5 to 7 minutes total.
4. Divide among 4 plates. Immediately add lemon juice, the remaining ¼ teaspoon salt, and asparagus to the pan and cook, stirring constantly, until the asparagus is coated and heated through, about 2 minutes.
5. Serve the asparagus with the fish.

Nutrition:

- Calories: 211
- Fat: 10 g
- Carbs: 8 g
- Protein: 26 g
- Sugars: 0.4 g
- Sodium: 375.7 mg

Parmesan-Crusted Fish

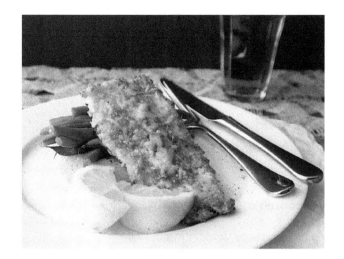

Preparation Time: 5 minutes

Cooking Time: 7 minutes

Servings: 2

Ingredients:

- ¾ tsp. ground ginger
- 1/3 c. panko bread crumbs
- Mixed fresh salad greens
- ¼ c. finely shredded parmesan cheese
- 1 tbsp. butter
- 4 skinless cod fillets
- 3 c. julienned carrots

Directions:

1. Preheat oven to 450 oF. Lightly coat a baking sheet with nonstick cooking spray.
2. Rinse and pat dry fish; place on the baking sheet. Season with salt and pepper.
3. In a small bowl stir together crumbs and cheese; sprinkle on fish.
4. Bake, uncovered, 4 to 6 minutes for each 1/2-inch thickness of fish, until crumbs are golden and fish flakes easily when tested with a fork.
5. Meanwhile, in a large skillet bring 1/2 cup water to boiling; add carrots. Reduce heat.
6. Cook, covered, for 5 minutes. Uncover; cook 2 minutes more. Add butter and ginger; toss.
7. Serve fish and carrots with greens.

Nutrition:

- Calories: 216.4
- Fat: 10.1 g
- Carbs: 1.3 g
- Protein: 29.0 g
- Sugars: 0.1 g
- Sodium: 428.3 mg

Lemon Swordfish

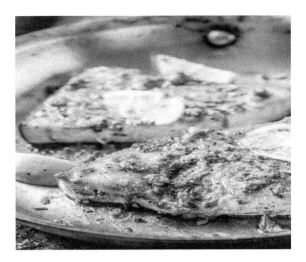

Preparation Time: 10 minutes

Cooking Time: 25 minutes

Servings: 2

Ingredients:

- 18 oz swordfish fillets
- 1 tablespoon margarine
- 1 teaspoon lemon zest
- 3 tablespoons lemon juice
- 1 teaspoon ground black pepper
- 2 tablespoons olive oil
- ½ teaspoon minced garlic

Directions:

1. Cut the fish into 4 servings.
2. After this, in the mixing bowl, mix up lemon zest, lemon juice, ground black pepper, and olive oil. Add minced garlic.
3. Rub the fish fillets with lemon mixture.
4. Grease the baking pan with margarine and arrange the swordfish fillets.
5. Bake the fish for 25 minutes at 390F.

Nutrition:

- 288 calories
- 32.6g protein
- 0.8g carbohydrates
- 16.5g fat
- 0.2g fiber
- 64mg cholesterol
- 183mg sodium

Spiced Scallops

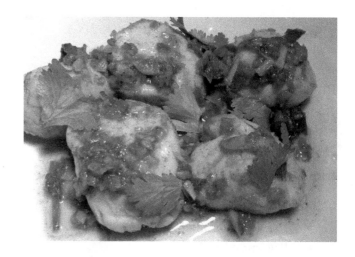

Preparation Time: 10 minutes

Cooking Time: 5 minutes

Servings: 2

Ingredients:

- 1-pound scallops
- 1 teaspoon Cajun seasonings
- 1 tablespoon olive oil

Directions:

1. Rub the scallops with Cajun seasonings.
2. Heat up olive oil in the skillet.
3. Add scallops and cook them for 2 minutes per each side.

Nutrition:

- 130 calories
- 19g protein
- 2.7g carbohydrates
- 4.4g fat
- 0g fiber
- 37mg cholesterol
- 195mg sodium

Shrimp Puttanesca

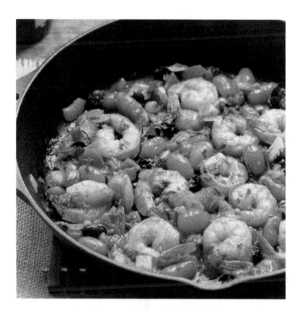

Preparation Time: 5 minutes

Cooking Time: 20 minutes

Servings: 2

Ingredients:

- 5 oz shrimps, peeled
- 1 teaspoon chili flakes
- ½ onion, diced
- 1 tablespoon coconut oil
- 1 teaspoon garlic, diced
- 1 cup tomatoes, chopped
- ¼ cup olives, sliced
- ¼ cup of water

Directions:

1. Heat up coconut oil in the saucepan.
2. Add shrimps and chili flakes. Cook the shrimps for 4 minutes.
3. Stir them well and add diced onion, garlic, tomatoes, olives, and water.
4. Close the lid and sauté the meal for 15 minutes.

Nutrition:

- 128 calories
- 11.7g protein
- 5.8g carbohydrates
- 6.7g fat
- 1.5g fiber
- 100mg cholesterol
- 217mg sodium

Curry Snapper

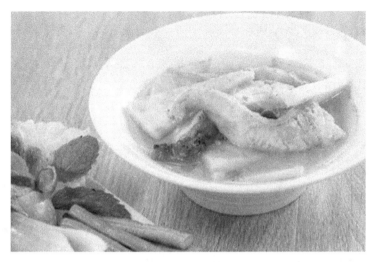

Preparation Time: 10 minutes

Cooking Time: 15 minutes

Servings: 2

Ingredients:

- 1-pound snapper fillet, chopped
- 1 teaspoon curry powder
- 1 cup celery stalk, chopped
- ½ cup low-fat yogurt
- ¼ cup of water
- 1 tablespoon olive oil

Directions:

1. Roast the snapper fillet in olive oil for 2 minutes per side.
2. Then add celery stalk, curry powder, low-fat yogurt, and water.
3. Stir the fish until you get the homogenous texture.
4. Close the lid and simmer the fish for 10 minutes on medium heat.

Nutrition:

- 195 calories
- 29.5g protein
- 3.2g carbohydrates
- 5.9g fat
- 0.6g fiber
- 52mg cholesterol
- 105mg sodium

Grouper with Tomato Sauce

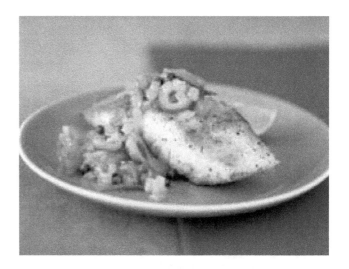

Preparation Time: 10 minutes

Cooking Time: 15 minutes

Servings: 2

Ingredients:

- 12 oz grouper, chopped
- 2 cups grape tomatoes, chopped
- 1 chili pepper, chopped
- 1 tablespoon margarine
- 1 teaspoon ground coriander

Directions:

1. Toss the margarine in the saucepan.
2. Add chopped grouper and sprinkle it with ground coriander.
3. Roast the fish for 2 minutes per side.
4. Then add grape tomatoes and chili pepper.
5. Stir the ingredients well and close the lid.
6. Cook the meal for 10 minutes on low heat.

Nutrition:

- 285 calories
- 43.9g protein
- 7.2g carbohydrates
- 8.3g fat
- 2.2g fiber
- 80mg cholesterol
- 166mg sodium

Braised Seabass

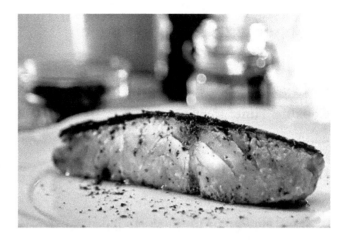

Preparation Time: 8 minutes

Cooking Time: 28 minutes

Servings: 2

Ingredients:

- 10 oz seabass fillet
- 1 cup tomatoes, chopped
- 1 yellow onion, sliced
- 1 tablespoon avocado oil
- 1 teaspoon ground black pepper

Directions:

1. Heat up olive oil in the skillet.
2. Add seabass fillet and roast it for 4 minutes per side.
3. Then remove the fish from the skillet and add sliced onion.
4. Cook it for 2 minutes.
5. After this, add tomatoes, and ground black pepper.
6. Bring the mixture to a boil.
7. Add cooked seabass and close the lid.
8. Cook the meal for 15 minutes.

Nutrition:

- 285 calories
- 27.7g protein
- 9.7g carbohydrates
- 15.3g fat
- 3.8g fiber
- 0mg cholesterol
- 8mg sodium

CHAPTER 21:

Pork & Beef

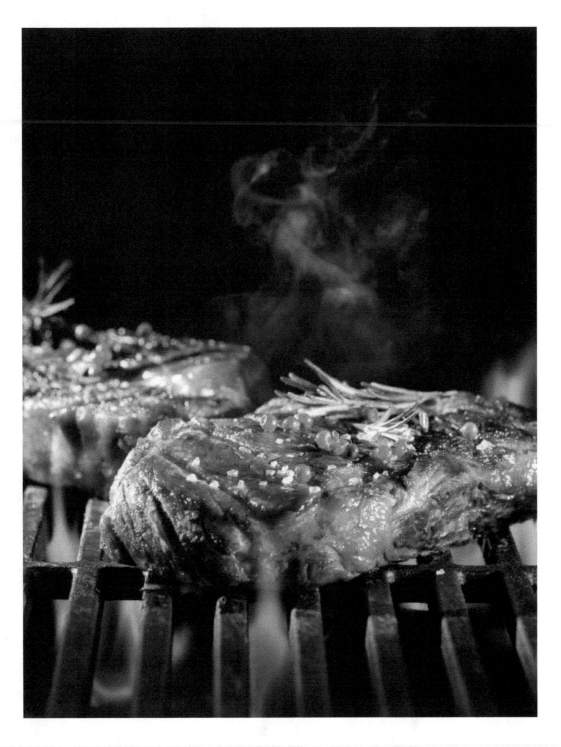

Beef Stroganoff

Preparation Time: 50 minutes

Cooking Time: 45 minutes

Servings: 2

Ingredients:

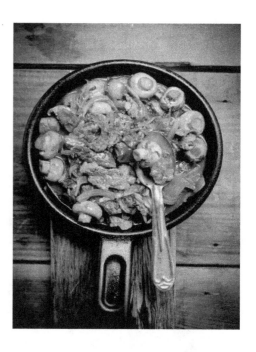

- One cup sour cream, fat-free
- Four cloves garlic, crushed
- Sixteen oz. fettuccine noodles, whole wheat
- One lb. mushrooms, sliced
- Four tbsp. margarine, separated
- One cup onion, chopped
- Two tbsp. whole wheat flour
- One and one-half lb. beef fillet steaks, lean
- Two tsp. Mustard, low-sodium
- One-half tsp. salt, separated
- Two cups vegetable broth, low-salt
- One tsp. paprika seasoning
- Three tsp. Worcestershire sauce, low-sodium
- One-half tsp. black pepper, separated
- Sixteen cups water
- One-third cup white wine, dry

Directions:

1. Prepare the onion by removing the skin and dicing it into small sections. Set aside.
2. Rub any extra dirt off of the mushrooms and slice. Set to the side.
3. Warm a deep pot with the water and the whole wheat fettuccine noodles with one-fourth teaspoon of the salt for approximately 10 minutes.
4. In the meantime, chop the beef into small cubes and dust with one-fourth teaspoon of pepper.
5. Liquefy two tablespoons of the margarine in a big skillet and transfer the cubed meat into the pan. Fry the meat for approximately 8 minutes while tossing occasionally to fully brown.
6. Remove the water from the cooked pasta and set to the side.
7. Use a spoon with holes to distribute the cooked meat to a platter and keep to the side.
8. Dissolve the leftover two tablespoons of margarine in the hot frying pan and fry the onions for approximately 5 minutes to caramelize.
9. Blend the garlic into the pan and heat for an additional half minute.
10. Then combine the mushrooms with the onions and fry for about 4 minutes.
11. Season the vegetables with the paprika and mustard and empty the wine into the skillet and heat for another 6 minutes, occasionally tossing and rubbing the base of the pan with a spatula that is wooden.
12. Meanwhile, blend the Worcestershire sauce, flour, and vegetable broth in a glass dish until there are no lumps present.

13. Empty the sauce into the skillet and bring to a slow bubble for approximately 5 minutes while occasionally stirring.
14. Transfer the cooked meat to the skillet and spice with the remaining one-fourth teaspoons of pepper and salt.
15. Turn the burner down to the setting of low and blend the sour cream into the skillet. Heat for an additional two minutes.
16. Distribute the cooked noodles into the pan and cover them fully with the sauce.
17. Spoon into serving dishes and enjoy immediately.

Nutrition:

- Sodium: 458 mg
- Protein: 42 g
- Fat: 11 g
- Sugar: 4 g
- Calories: 442

Pork Roast with Orange Sauce

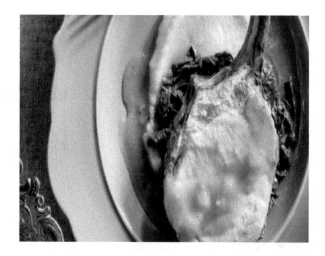

Preparation Time: 15 minutes

Cooking Time: 80 minutes

Servings: 2

Ingredients:

- 1-pound pork loin roast
- ½ cup carrot, diced
- ½ cup celery stalk, chopped
- ½ cup onion, diced
- 1 teaspoon Italian seasonings
- 1 cup of orange juice
- 1 tablespoon potato starch

Directions:

1. Rub the pork loin roast with Italian seasonings.
2. Then put the carrot, celery stalk, and diced onion in the tray.
3. Put the meat over the vegetables. Add orange juice.
4. Bake the meat for 75 minutes at 365F.
5. After this, transfer all vegetables and juice to the saucepan and bring it to a boil.
6. Blend the mixture with the help of the blender. Add potato starch and whisk it well.
7. Simmer the sauce for 2 minutes.
8. Slice the cooked meat and sprinkle it with orange sauce.

Nutrition:

- 292 calories
- 33.2g protein
- 12.2g carbohydrates
- 11.4g fat
- 1g fiber
- 93mg cholesterol
- 87mg sodium

Southwestern Steak

Preparation Time: 15 minutes

Cooking Time: 16 minutes

Servings: 2

Ingredients:

- 2 beef flank steaks
- 1 tablespoon lemon juice
- 1 teaspoon chili flakes
- 1 teaspoon garlic powder
- 1 tablespoon avocado oil

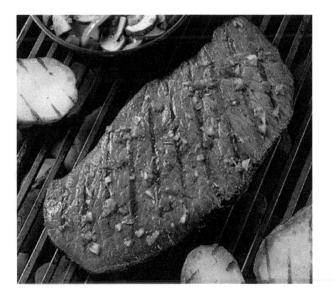

Directions:

1. Preheat the grill to 385F.
2. Then rub the meat with chili flakes and garlic powder.
3. Then sprinkle it with lemon juice and avocado oil.
4. Grill the steaks for 8 minutes per side.

Nutrition:

- 174 calories
- 26.2g protein
- 1.6g carbohydrates
- 6.3g fat
- 0.5g fiber
- 76mg cholesterol
- 58mg sodium

Tender Pork Medallions

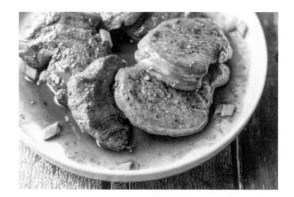

Preparation Time: 10 minutes

Cooking Time: 25 minutes

Servings: 2

Ingredients:

- 12 oz pork tenderloin
- 1 teaspoon dried sage
- 1 tablespoon margarine
- 1 teaspoon ground black pepper
- ½ cup low-fat yogurt

Directions:

1. Cut the pork tenderloin into 3 medallions and sprinkle with sage and ground black pepper.
2. Heat up margarine in the saucepan and add pork medallions.
3. Roast them for 5 minutes per side.
4. Then add yogurt and coat the meat in it well.
5. Close the lid and simmer the medallions for 15 minutes over medium heat.

Nutrition:

- 227 calories
- 32.4g protein
- 3.5g carbohydrates
- 8.3g fat
- 0.3g fiber
- 85mg cholesterol
- 138mg sodium

Garlic Pork Meatballs

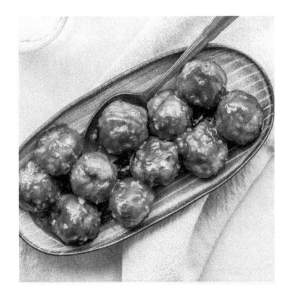

Preparation Time: 10 minutes

Cooking Time: 28 minutes

Servings: 2

Ingredients:

- 2 pork medallions
- 1 teaspoon minced garlic
- ¼ cup of coconut milk
- 1 tablespoon olive oil
- 1 teaspoon cayenne pepper

Directions:

1. Sprinkle each pork medallion with cayenne pepper.
2. Heat up olive oil in the skillet and add meat.
3. Roast the pork medallions for 3 minutes from each side.
4. After this, add coconut milk and minced garlic. Close the lid and simmer the meat for 20 minutes on low heat.

Nutrition:

- 284 calories
- 25.9g protein
- 2.6g carbohydrates
- 18.8g fat
- 0.9g fiber
- 70mg cholesterol
- 60mg sodium

Fajita Pork Strips

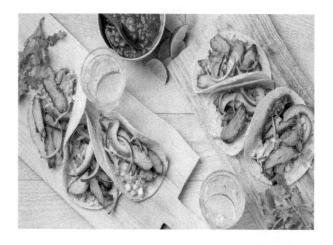

Preparation Time: 10 minutes

Cooking Time: 35 minutes

Servings: 2

Ingredients:

- 16 oz pork sirloin
- 1 tablespoon Fajita seasonings
- 1 tablespoon canola oil

Directions:

1. Cut the pork sirloin into strips and sprinkle with fajita seasonings and canola oil.
2. Then transfer the meat to the baking tray in one layer.
3. Bake it for 35 minutes at 365F. Stir the meat every 10 minutes during cooking.

Nutrition:

- 184 calories
- 18.5g protein
- 1.3g carbohydrates
- 10.8g fat
- 0g fiber
- 64mg cholesterol
- 157mg sodium

Pepper Pork Tenderloins

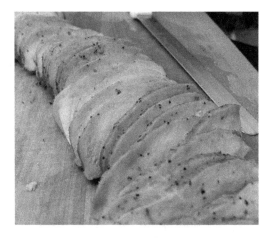

Preparation Time: 15 minutes

Cooking Time: 60 minutes

Servings: 2

Ingredients:

- 8 oz pork tenderloin
- 1 tablespoon mustard
- 1 teaspoon ground black pepper
- 2 tablespoons olive oil

Directions:

1. Rub the meat with mustard and sprinkle with ground black pepper.
2. Then brush it with olive oil and wrap it in the foil.
3. Bake the meat for 60 minutes at 375F.
4. Then discard the foil and slice the tenderloin into servings.

Nutrition:

- 311 calories
- 31.2g protein
- 2.6g carbohydrates
- 19.6g fat
- 1.1g fiber
- 83mg cholesterol
- 65mg sodium

Spiced Beef

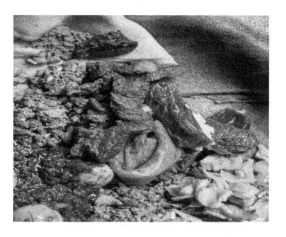

Preparation Time: 10 minutes

Cooking Time: 80 minutes

Servings: 2

Ingredients:

- 1-pound beef sirloin
- 1 tablespoon five-spice seasoning
- 1 bay leaf
- 2 cups of water
- 1 teaspoon peppercorn

Directions:

1. Rub the meat with five-spice seasoning and put it in the saucepan.
2. Add nay leaf, water, and peppercorns.
3. Close the lid and simmer it for 80 minutes on medium heat.
4. Chop the cooked meat and sprinkle it with hot spiced water from the saucepan.

Nutrition:

- 213 calories
- 34.5g protein
- 0.5g carbohydrates
- 7.1g fat
- 0.2g fiber
- 101mg cholesterol
- 116mg sodium

Tomato Beef

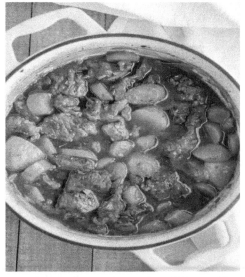

Preparation Time: 10 minutes

Cooking Time: 17 minutes

Servings: 2

Ingredients:

- 2 chuck shoulder steaks
- ¼ cup tomato sauce
- 1 tablespoon olive oil

Directions:

1. Brush the steaks with tomato sauce and olive oil and transfer to the preheated to 390F grill.
2. Grill the meat for 9 minutes.
3. Then flip it on another side and cook for 8 minutes more.

Nutrition:

- 247 calories
- 21.4g protein
- 1.7g carbohydrates
- 17.1g fat
- 0.5g fiber
- 70mg cholesterol
- 231mg sodium

Hoisin Pork

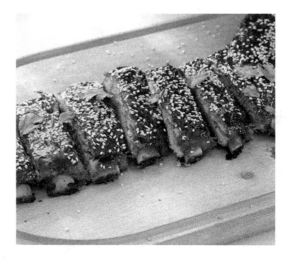

Preparation Time: 10 minutes

Cooking Time: 14 minutes

Servings: 2

Ingredients:

- 1-pound pork loin steaks
- 2 tablespoons hoisin sauce
- 1 tablespoon apple cider vinegar
- 1 teaspoon olive oil

Directions:

1. Rub the pork steaks with hoisin sauce, apple cider vinegar, and olive oil.
2. Then preheat the grill to 395F.
3. Put the pork steak in the grill and cook them for 7 minutes per side.

Nutrition:

- 263 calories
- 39.3g protein
- 3.6g carbohydrates
- 10.1g fat
- 0.2g fiber
- 0mg cholesterol
- 130mg sodium

Sage Beef Loin

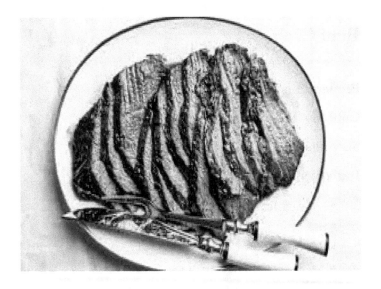

Preparation Time: 10 minutes

Cooking Time: 18 minutes

Servings: 2

Ingredients:

- 10 oz beef loin, strips
- 1 garlic clove, diced
- 2 tablespoons margarine
- 1 teaspoon dried sage

Directions:

1. Toss margarine in the skillet.
2. Add garlic and dried sage and roast them for 2 minutes on low heat.
3. Add beef loin strips and roast them for 15 minutes on medium heat. Stir the meat occasionally.

Nutrition:

- 363 calories
- 38.2g protein
- 0.8g carbohydrates
- 23.2g fat
- 0.2g fiber
- 101mg cholesterol
- 211mg sodium

Beef Chili

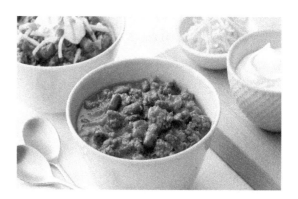

Preparation Time: 10 minutes

Cooking Time: 30 minutes

Servings: 2

Ingredients:

- 1 cup lean ground beef
- 1 onion, diced
- 1 tablespoon olive oil
- 1 cup crushed tomatoes
- ½ cup red kidney beans, cooked
- ½ cup of water
- 1 teaspoon chili seasonings

Directions:

1. Heat up olive oil in the saucepan and add lean ground beef.
2. Cook it for 7 minutes over medium heat.
3. Then add chili seasonings and diced onion. Stir the ingredients and cook them for 10 minutes.
4. After this, add water, crushed tomatoes, red kidney beans, and stir the chili well.
5. Close the lid and simmer the meal for 13 minutes.

Nutrition:

- 220 calories
- 18.3g protein
- 22g carbohydrates
- 6.7g fat
- 6.1g fiber
- 34mg cholesterol
- 177mg sodium

Celery Beef Stew

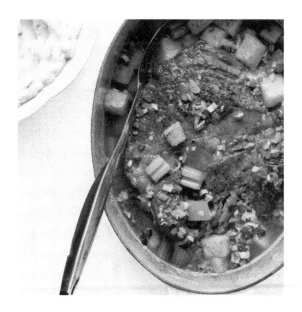

Preparation Time: 5 minutes

Cooking Time: 55 minutes

Servings: 2

Ingredients:

- 1-pound beef loin, chopped
- 2 cups celery stalk, chopped
- 1 garlic clove, diced
- 1 yellow onion, diced
- 1 tablespoon olive oil
- 1 tablespoon tomato paste
- 1 teaspoon chili powder
- 1 teaspoon dried dill
- 2 cups of water

Directions:

1. Roast the beef loin with olive oil in the saucepan for 5 minutes.
2. After this, add all remaining ingredients and close the lid.
3. Cook the stew for 50 minutes on medium heat.

Nutrition:

- 150 calories
- 14.6g protein
- 4.6g carbohydrates
- 7.9g fat
- 1.2g fiber
- 41mg cholesterol
- 370mg sodium

Beef Skillet

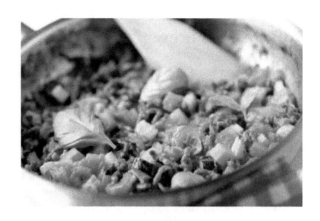

Preparation Time: 10 minutes

Cooking Time: 30 minutes

Servings: 2

Ingredients:

- 1 cup lean ground beef
- 1 cup bell pepper, sliced
- 2 tomatoes, chopped
- 1 chili pepper, chopped
- 1 tablespoon olive oil
- ½ cup of water

Directions:

1. Heat up olive oil in the skillet and add lean ground beef.
2. Roast it for 10 minutes.
3. Then stir the meat well and add chili pepper and bell pepper. Roast the ingredients for 10 minutes more.
4. Add tomatoes and water.
5. Close the lid and simmer the meal for 10 minutes.

Nutrition:

- 167 calories
- 16.1g protein
- 6.3g carbohydrates
- 8.8g fat
- 1.6g fiber
- 46mg cholesterol
- 50mg sodium

Hot Beef Strips

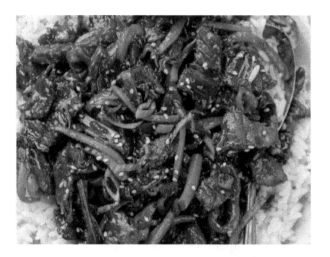

Preparation Time: 10 minutes

Cooking Time: 15 minutes

Servings: 2

Ingredients:

- 9 oz beef tenders
- 2 tablespoons cayenne pepper
- 1 tablespoon lemon juice
- 2 tablespoons canola oil

Directions:

1. Cut the beef tenders into strips and rub with cayenne pepper.
2. Sprinkle the meat with lemon juice and put it in the hot skillet.
3. Add canola oil and roast the meat for 15 minutes on medium heat. Stir it from time to time to avoid burning.

Nutrition:

- 231 calories
- 22.5g protein
- 2.1g carbohydrates
- 14.6g fat
- 1g fiber
- 54mg cholesterol
- 62mg sodium

Sloppy Joe

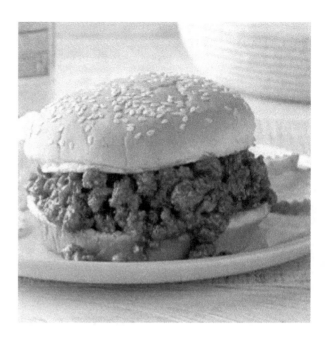

Preparation Time: 10 minutes

Cooking Time: 35 minutes

Servings: 2

Ingredients:

- 1 cup lean ground beef
- 1 cup onion, diced
- ½ cup sweet peppers, diced
- 1 teaspoon minced garlic
- 1 tablespoon canola oil
- 1 teaspoon liquid honey
- ½ cup tomato puree
- 1 teaspoon tomato paste

Directions:

1. Mix up canola oil and lean ground beef in the saucepan.
2. Add onion and sweet pepper and stir the ingredient well.
3. Cook them for 10 minutes.
4. Then add honey, tomato puree, and tomato paste. Mix up the mixture well.
5. Close the lid and cook it for 25 minutes on medium heat.

Nutrition:

- 134 calories
- 7.6g protein
- 8.7g carbohydrates
- 7.7g fat
- 1.9g fiber
- 22mg cholesterol
- 34mg sodium

CHAPTER 22:

Snacks, Sides & Desserts

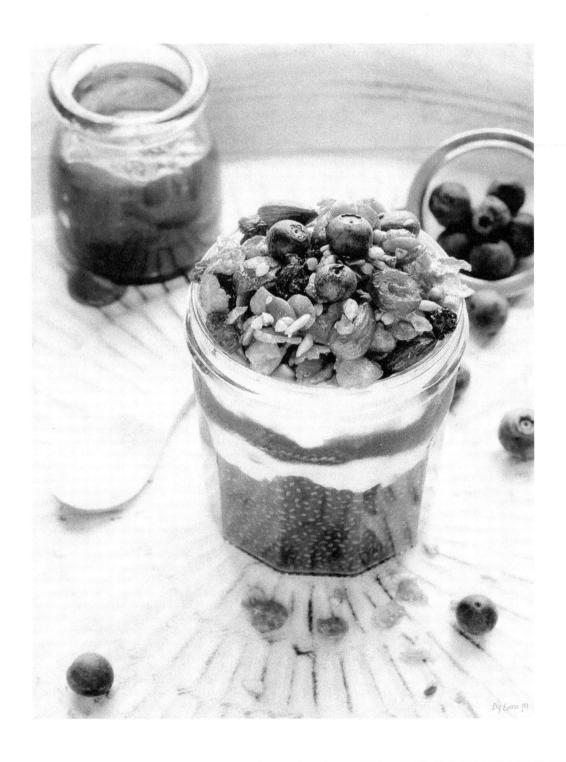

Summer Squash Ribbons with Lemon and Ricotta

Preparation Time: 20 minutes

Cooking Time: 0 minutes

Servings: 2

Ingredients:

- 2 medium zucchini or yellow squash
- ½ cup ricotta cheese
- 2 tablespoons fresh mint, chopped, plus additional mint leaves for garnish
- 2 tablespoons fresh parsley, chopped
- Zest of ½ lemon
- 2 teaspoons lemon juice
- ½ teaspoon kosher salt
- ¼ teaspoon freshly ground black pepper
- 1 tablespoon extra-virgin olive oil

Directions:

1. Using a vegetable peeler, make ribbons by peeling the summer squash lengthwise. The squash ribbons will resemble the wide pasta, pappardelle.
2. In a medium bowl, combine the ricotta cheese, mint, parsley, lemon zest, lemon juice, salt, and black pepper.
3. Place mounds of the squash ribbons evenly on 4 plates then dollop the ricotta mixture on top. Drizzle with olive oil and garnish with the mint leaves.

Nutrition:

- Calories: 90
- Total Fat: 6g
- Cholesterol: 10mg
- Sodium: 180mg
- Total Carbohydrates: 5g
- Fiber: 1g
- Sugars: 3g
- Protein: 5g

Sautéed Kale with Tomato and Garlic

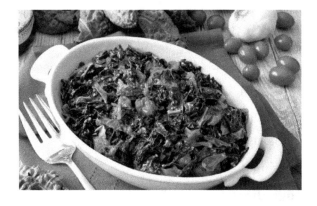

Preparation Time: 5 minutes

Cooking Time: 10 minutes

Servings: 1

Ingredients:

- 1 tablespoon extra-virgin olive oil
- 4 garlic cloves, sliced
- ¼ teaspoon red pepper flakes
- 2 bunches kale, stemmed and chopped or torn into pieces
- 1 (14.5-ounce) can no-salt-added diced tomatoes
- ½ teaspoon kosher salt

Directions:

1. Heat the olive oil in a wok or large skillet over medium-high heat. Add the garlic and red pepper flakes, and sauté until fragrant, about 30 seconds. Add the kale and sauté, about 3 to 5 minutes, until the kale shrinks down a bit.
2. Add the tomatoes and the salt, stir together, and cook for 3 to 5 minutes, or until the liquid reduces and the kale cooks down further and becomes tender.

Nutrition:

- Calories: 110
- Total Fat: 5g
- Cholesterol: 0mg
- Sodium: 222mg
- Total Carbohydrates: 15g
- Fiber: 6g
- Sugars: 6g
- Protein: 6g

Roasted Broccoli with Tahini Yogurt Sauce

Preparation Time: 15 minutes

Cooking Time: 30 minutes

Servings: 2

Ingredients:

- 1½ to 2 pounds broccoli, stalk trimmed and cut into slices, head cut into florets
- 1 lemon, sliced into ¼-inch-thick rounds
- 3 tablespoons extra-virgin olive oil
- ½ teaspoon kosher salt
- ¼ teaspoon freshly ground black pepper
- ½ cup plain Greek yogurt
- 2 tablespoons tahini
- 1 tablespoon lemon juice
- ¼ teaspoon kosher salt
- 1 teaspoon sesame seeds, for garnish (optional)

Directions:

1. Preheat the oven to 425°F. Line a baking sheet with parchment paper or foil.
2. In a large bowl, gently toss the broccoli, lemon slices, olive oil, salt, and black pepper to combine. Arrange the broccoli in a single layer on the prepared baking sheet. Roast 15 minutes, stir, and roast another 15 minutes, until golden brown.

To Make The Tahini Yogurt Sauce:

1. In a medium bowl, combine the yogurt, tahini, lemon juice, and salt; mix well.
2. Spread the tahini yogurt sauce on a platter or large plate and top with the broccoli and lemon slices. Garnish with the sesame seeds (if desired).

Nutrition:

- Calories: 245
- Total Fat: 16g
- Cholesterol: 2mg
- Sodium: 305mg
- Total Carbohydrates: 20g
- Fiber: 7g
- Sugars: 6g
- Protein: 12g

Green Beans with Pine Nuts and Garlic

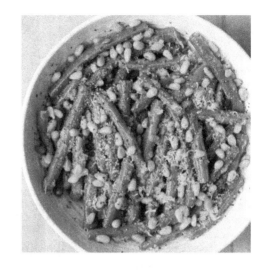

Preparation Time: 10 minutes

Cooking Time: 20 minutes

Servings: 1-2

Ingredients:

- 1 pound green beans, trimmed
- 1 head garlic (10 to 12 cloves), smashed
- 2 tablespoons extra-virgin olive oil
- ½ teaspoon kosher salt
- ¼ teaspoon red pepper flakes
- 1 tablespoon white wine vinegar
- ¼ cup pine nuts, toasted

Directions:

1. Preheat the oven to 425°F. Line a baking sheet with parchment paper or foil.
2. In a large bowl, combine the green beans, garlic, olive oil, salt, and red pepper flakes and mix. Arrange in a single layer on the baking sheet. Roast for 10 minutes, stir, and roast for another 10 minutes, or until golden brown.
3. Mix the cooked green beans with the vinegar and top with the pine nuts.

Nutrition:

- Calories: 165
- Total Fat: 13g
- Cholesterol: 0mg
- Sodium: 150mg
- Total Carbohydrates: 12g
- Fiber: 4g
- Sugars: 4g
- Protein: 4g

Roasted Harissa Carrots

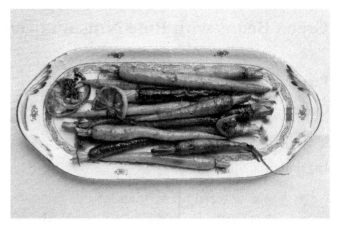

Preparation Time: 10 minutes

Cooking Time: 15 minutes

Servings: 2

Ingredients:

- 1 pound carrots, peeled and sliced into 1-inch-thick rounds
- 2 tablespoons extra-virgin olive oil
- 2 tablespoons harissa
- 1 teaspoon honey
- 1 teaspoon ground cumin
- ½ teaspoon kosher salt
- ½ cup fresh parsley, chopped

Directions:

1. Preheat the oven to 450°F. Line a baking sheet with parchment paper or foil.
2. In a large bowl, combine the carrots, olive oil, harissa, honey, cumin, and salt. Arrange in a single layer on the baking sheet. Roast for 15 minutes. Remove from the oven, add the parsley, and toss together.

Nutrition:

- Calories: 120
- Total Fat: 8g
- Cholesterol: 0mg
- Sodium: 255mg
- Total Carbohydrates: 13g
- Fiber: 4g
- Sugars: 7g
- Protein: 1g

Toasted Almond Ambrosia

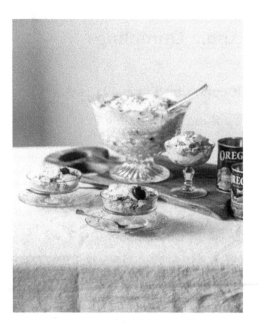

Preparation Time: 30 minutes

Cooking Time: 0 minutes

Servings: 2

Ingredients:

- ½ cup almonds, slivered
- ½ cup coconut, shredded & unsweetened
- 3 cups pineapple, cubed
- 5 oranges, cut
- 1 banana, halved lengthwise, peeled & sliced
- 2 red apples, cored & diced
- 2 tablespoons cream sherry
- mint leaves, fresh to garnish

Directions:

1. Start by heating your oven to 325, and then get out a baking sheet. Roast your almonds for ten minutes, making sure they're spread out evenly.
2. Transfer them to a plate and then toast your coconut on the same baking sheet. Toast for ten minutes.
3. Mix your banana, sherry, oranges, apples, and pineapple in a bowl.
4. Divide the mixture not serving bowls and top with coconut and almonds.
5. Garnish with mint before serving.

Nutrition:

- Calories: 177
- Protein: 3.4 g
- Fat: 4.9 g
- Carbs: 36 g
- Sodium: 13 mg
- Cholesterol: 11 mg

Apple Dumplings

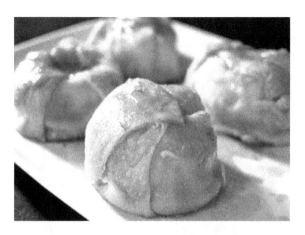

Preparation Time: 40 minutes

Cooking Time: 0 minutes

Servings: 2

Ingredients:

Dough:

- 1 tablespoon butter
- 1 teaspoon honey, raw
- 1 cup whole wheat flour
- 2 tablespoons buckwheat flour
- 2 tablespoons rolled oats
- 2 tablespoons brandy or apple liquor

Filling:

- 2 tablespoons honey, raw
- 1 teaspoon nutmeg
- 6 tart apples, sliced thin
- 1 lemon, zested

Directions:

1. Turn the oven to 350. Get out a food processor and mix your butter, flours, honey, and oats until it forms a crumbly mixture. Add in your brandy or apple liquor, pulsing until it forms a dough.
2. Seal in plastic and place it in the fridge for two hours.
3. Toss your apples in lemon zest, honey, and nutmeg.
4. Roll your dough into a sheet that's a quarter-inch thick. Cut out eight-inch circles, placing each circle into a muffin tray that's been greased.
5. Press the dough down and then stuff with the apple mixture. Fold the edges, and pinch them closed. Make sure that they're well sealed.
6. Bake for a half-hour until golden brown, and serve drizzled in honey.

Nutrition:

- Calories: 178
- Protein: 5 g
- Fat: 4 g
- Carbs: 23 g
- Sodium: 562 mg
- Cholesterol: 61 mg

Almond Rice Pudding

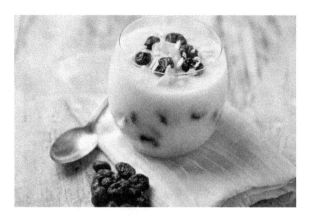

Preparation Time: 25 minutes

Cooking Time: 20 minutes

Servings: 2

Ingredients:

- 3 cups 1% milk
- 1 cup white rice
- 1⁄4 cup sugar
- 1 teaspoon vanilla
- 1⁄4 teaspoon almond extract
- Cinnamon
- 1⁄4 cup toasted almonds

Directions:

1. Combine milk and rice in a medium saucepan. Bring them to a boil.
2. Reduce heat and simmer for 20 minutes with the lid on until the rice is soft.
3. Remove from heat and add the sugar, vanilla, almond extract, and cinnamon.
4. Sprinkle toasted almonds on top and serve warm.

Nutrition:

- Calories 180
- Total fat 1.5 g
- Carbohydrates 36 g
- Protein 7 g
- Fiber 1 g
- Sodium 65 mg

Apples and Cream Shake

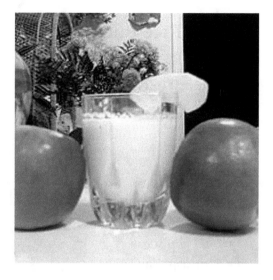

Preparation Time: 10 minutes

Cooking Time: 0 minutes

Servings: 1

Ingredients:

- 2 cups vanilla low fat ice cream
- 1 cup apple sauce
- 1/4 teaspoon ground cinnamon
- 1 cup fat-free skim milk

Directions:

1. In a blender container combine the low-fat ice cream, applesauce, and cinnamon. Cover and blend until smooth.
2. Add fat-free skim milk. Cover and blend until mixed.
3. Pour into glasses.
4. Serve immediately.

Nutrition:

- Calories 160
- Total fat 3 g
- Carbohydrates 27 g
- Protein 6 g
- Fiber 1 g
- Sodium 80 mg

Baked Stuffed Apples

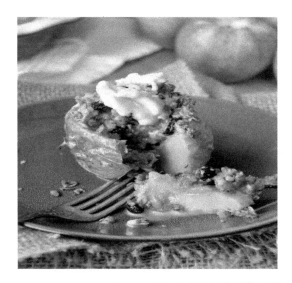

Preparation Time: 10 minutes

Cooking Time: 8 minutes

Servings: 2

Ingredients:

- 4 Jonagold apples
- 1/4 cup flaked coconut
- 1/4 cup chopped dried apricots
- 2 teaspoons grated orange zest
- 1/2 cup orange juice
- 2 tablespoons brown sugar

Directions:

1. Peel top 1/3 of apples and hollow out center with a knife. Arrange, peeled end up, in a microwave-safe baking dish. Combine coconut, apricots, and orange zest. Divide to evenly fill centers of apples.
2. Mix orange juice and brown sugar. Pour over apples. Cover tightly with vented plastic wrap and microwave on high for 8 minutes or until apples are tender. Cool before serving.

Nutrition:

- Calories 192
- Total fat 2 g
- Carbohydrates 46 g
- Protein 1 g
- Fiber 6 g
- Sodium 19 mg

Apricot Biscotti

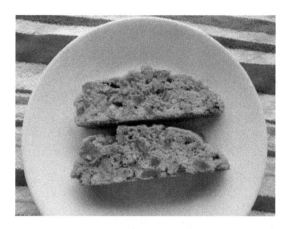

Preparation Time: 50 minutes

Cooking Time: 0 minutes

Servings: 2

Ingredients:

- 2 tablespoons honey, dark
- 2 tablespoons olive oil
- ½ teaspoon almond extract
- ¼ cup almonds, chopped roughly
- 2/3 cup apricots, dried
- 2 tablespoons milk, 1% & low fat
- 2 eggs, beaten lightly
- ¾ cup whole wheat flour
- ¾ cup all-purpose flour
- ¼ cup brown sugar, packed firm
- 1 teaspoon baking powder

Directions:

1. Start by heating the oven to 350, and then mix your baking powder, brown sugar, and flours in a bowl.
2. Whisk your canola oil, eggs, almond extract, honey, and milk. Mix well until it forms a smooth dough. Fold in the apricots and almonds.
3. Put your dough on plastic wrap, and then roll it out to a twelve-inch long and three-inch wide rectangle. Place this dough on a baking sheet, and bake for twenty-five minutes. It should turn golden brown. Allow it to cool, and slice it into ½ inch thick slices, and then bake for another fifteen minutes. It should be crispy.

Nutrition:

- Calories: 291
- Protein: 2 g
- Fat: 2 g
- Carbs: 12 g
- Sodium: 123 mg
- Cholesterol: 21 mg

Apple & Berry Cobbler

Preparation Time: 40minutes

Cooking Time: 0 minutes

Servings: 2

Ingredients:

Filling:

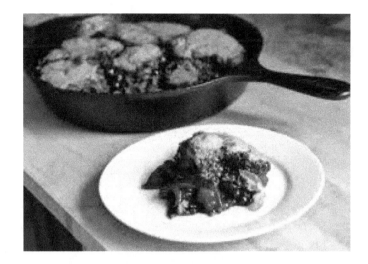

- 1 cup blueberries, fresh
- 2 cups apples, chopped
- 1 cup raspberries, fresh
- 2 tablespoons brown sugar
- 1 teaspoon lemon zest
- 2 teaspoon lemon juice, fresh
- ½ teaspoon ground cinnamon
- 1 ½ tablespoons corn starch

Topping:

- ¾ cup whole wheat pastry flour
- 1 ½ tablespoons brown sugar
- ½ teaspoon vanilla extract, pure
- ¼ cup soy milk
- ¼ teaspoon sea salt, fine
- 1 egg white

Directions:

1. Turn your oven to 350, and get out six small ramekins. Grease them with cooking spray. Mix your lemon juice, lemon zest, blueberries, sugar, cinnamon, raspberries, and apples together in a bowl.
2. Stir in your cornstarch, mixing until it dissolves.
3. Beat your egg white in a different bowl, whisking it with sugar, vanilla, soy milk, and pastry flour.
4. Divide your berry mixture between the ramekins and top with the vanilla topping.
5. Put your ramekins on a baking sheet, baking for thirty minutes. The top should be golden brown before serving.

Nutrition:

- Calories: 131 Protein: 7.2 g
- Fat: 1 g Carbs: 13.8 g Sodium: 14 mg Cholesterol: 2.1 mg

Mixed Fruit Compote Cups

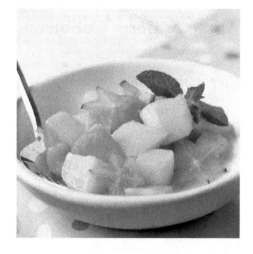

Preparation Time: 15minutes

Cooking Time: 0 minutes

Servings: 2

Ingredients:

- 1 ¼ cup water
- ½ cup orange juice
- 12 ounces mixed dried fruit
- 1 teaspoon ground cinnamon
- ¼ teaspoon ground ginger
- ¼ teaspoon ground nutmeg
- 4 cups vanilla frozen yogurt, fat-free

Directions:

1. Mix your dried fruit, nutmeg, cinnamon, water, orange juice, and ginger in a saucepan.
2. Cover, and allow it to cook over medium heat for ten minutes. Remove the cover, and then cook for another ten minutes.
3. Add your frozen yogurt to serving cups, and top with the fruit mixture.

Nutrition:

- Calories: 228
- Protein: 9.1 g
- Fat: 5.7 g
- Carbs: 12.4 g
- Sodium: 114 mg
- Cholesterol: 15 mg

Oatmeal Surprise Cookies

Preparation Time: 25minutes

Cooking Time: 0 minutes

Servings: 2

Ingredients:

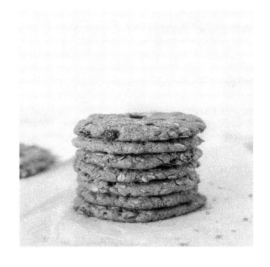

- 1 ½ cups creamy peanut butter, all natural
- ½ cup dark brown sugar
- 2 eggs, large
- 1 cup old fashioned rolled oats
- 1 teaspoon baking soda
- ½ teaspoon sea salt, fine
- ½ cup dark chocolate chips

Directions:

1. Start by heating your oven to 350, and get out a baking sheet. Line your baking sheet with parchment paper.
2. Get out a bowl with an electric mixer and whip your peanut butter until smooth. Continue beating as you add in your brown sugar. Keep beating as you add in one egg at a time until it's incorporated and fluffy. Beat in your oats, salt, and baking soda. Turn the mixer off and fold in your dark chocolate chips.
3. Put your cookie dough on a baking sheet two inches apart and bake for eight to ten minutes.

Nutrition:

- Calories: 152
- Protein: 4 g
- Fat: 10 g
- Carbs: 12 g
- Sodium: 131 mg
- Cholesterol: 18 mg

Almond & Apricot Crisp

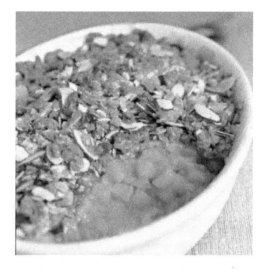

Preparation Time: 35 minutes

Cooking Time: 0 minutes

Servings: 2

Ingredients:

- 1 teaspoon olive oil
- 1 lb. Apricot, halved & pits removed
- ½ cup almonds, chopped
- 1 tablespoons oats
- 1 teaspoon anise seeds
- 2 tablespoons honey, raw

Directions:

1. Start by heating the oven to 350, and then grease a nine-inch pie plate with olive oil.
2. Add in your apricots once they're chopped, and spread them out evenly.
3. Top with anise seeds, oats, and almonds. Pour honey on top, and bake for twenty-five minutes. It should turn golden brown.

Nutrition:

- Calories: 149
- Protein: 3 g
- Fat: 11.9 g
- Carbs: 18.8 g
- Sodium: 79 mg
- Cholesterol: 78 mg

Blueberry Apple Cobbler

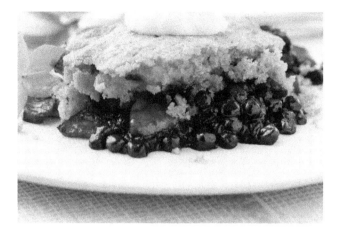

Preparation Time: 40 minutes

Cooking Time: 0 minutes

Servings: 2

Ingredients:

- 2 tablespoons cornstarch
- 2 tablespoons sugar
- 1 tablespoon lemon juice, fresh
- 2 apples, large, peeled, cored & sliced
- 1 teaspoon ground cinnamon
- 12 ounces blueberries, fresh

Toppings:

- ¼ teaspoon sea salt, fine
- ¾ cup all-purpose flour
- ¾ cup whole wheat flour
- 2 tablespoons sugar
- 1 ½ teaspoons baking powder
- 4 tablespoons margarine, cold & chopped
- ½ cup milk, fat-free
- 1 teaspoon vanilla extract, pure

Directions:

1. Turn the oven to 400 degrees, and then get out a nine-inch baking pan. Grease it using cooking spray. Mix your lemon juice and apples in a bowl before adding in your cornstarch, sugar, and cinnamon. Make sure it's evenly coated.
2. Toss the blueberries in, and then spread the mixture into the baking dish.
3. Get out a bowl and mix baking powder, both flours, sugar, and salt together.
4. Cut the margarine and mix it in until it forms a crumbly dough.
5. Stir in the milk and vanilla, and mix well to form a moist dough.
6. Knead with floured hands. Roll it out into a half an inch-thick rectangle.
7. Cut the dough into your favorite shapes using a cookie cutter.
8. Use the remaining scraps to cut more cookies.
9. Place this on top of your apple mixture until it is completely covered, and bake for a half-hour before serving.

Nutrition:

- Calories: 288 Protein: 6 g Fat: 6.2 g Carbs: 48 g Sodium: 176 mg
- Cholesterol: 120 mg

CHAPTER 23:

Measurement Conversions

Measurement

Cup	Ounces	Milliliters	Tablespoons
8 cups	64 oz	1895 ml	128
6 cups	48 oz	1420 ml	96
5 cups	40 oz	1180 ml	80
4 cups	32 oz	960 ml	64
2 cups	16 oz	480 ml	32
1 cup	8 oz	240 ml	16
3/4 cup	6 oz	177 ml	12
2/3 cup	5 oz	158 ml	11
1/2 cup	4 oz	118 ml	8
3/8 cup	3 oz	90 ml	6
1/3 cup	2.5 oz	79 ml	5.5
1/4 cup	2 oz	59 ml	4
1/8 cup	1 oz	30 ml	3
1/16 cup	1/2 oz	15 ml	1

Weight

Imperial	Metric
1/2 oz	15 g
1 oz	29 g
2 oz	57 g
3 oz	85 g
4 oz	113 g
5 oz	141 g
6 oz	170 g
8 oz	227 g
10 oz	283 g
12 oz	340 g
13 oz	369 g
14 oz	397 g
15 oz	425 g
1 lb	453 g

Temperature

Fahrenheit	Celsius
100 °F	37 °C
150 °F	65 °C
200 °F	93 °C
250 °F	121 °C
300 °F	150 °C
325 °F	160 °C
350 °F	180 °C
375 °F	190 °C
400 °F	200 °C
425 °F	220 °C
450 °F	230 °C
500 °F	260 °C
525 °F	274 °C
550 °F	288 °C

Conclusion

Statistics have it that one in three people have hypertension in America, and those that have normal blood pressure at the age of 50 or so have a 90% chance of getting affected in the near future. This is a high number considering how dangerous to your health hypertension can be. Having hypertension also means that you are prone to other health-related illnesses and diseases and this means an unhealthy life, and sometimes a short life.

This is not something that you cannot avoid though because making the right dietary choices has been seen to work really well to improve the health of people as well as reduce chances of suffering from hypertension and other health-related issues. The right choices can also make the existing condition manageable and you can still enjoy a longer, healthier life thereafter.

It is not too late to venture into a DASH Diet, a diet plan that will bring major changes in your health and life in general. This, along with staying active, limiting alcohol consumption, controlling your body weight, and staying stress-free will help a lot in enjoying a long happy life.

DASH diet is very easy to follow as it is the easiest diet plan so far but if you have to make huge diet changes. In order to fully adapt the DASH diet in your life, it is good to start making small changes bit by bit. Replace some of the unhealthy foods with healthy foods one day at a time. It will not be hard to stick to the diet plan this way. Convince your mind that healthy foods are the right foods to eat at all times and always have these healthy foods at your disposal in the place of unhealthy ones.

CPSIA information can be obtained
at www.ICGtesting.com
Printed in the USA
LVHW100322120121
676231LV00009B/383